Elizabeth Stuckey

Type 2 Diabetes Recipes

71 Healthy And Quick Recipes For First Dishes, Main Courses And Desserts Low In Carbohydrates To Live A More Relaxed And Serene Life With A Daily Diet Plan

© Copyright 2021 by **Elizabeth Stuckey**

Table of Contents

Sweets and Desserts for Diabetics..77

Preface

The following indications have an EXCLUSIVE informative purpose and are not intended to replace the opinion of professional figures such as doctors, nutritionists or dieticians, whose intervention is necessary for the prescription and composition of PERSONALIZED food therapies.

Chapter 1 - Type 2 Diabetes Mellitus

Diabetes Mellitus Type 2 is a disease that affects glucose metabolism; if left untreated, this form of diabetes also affects the state of health, lowering the quality and life expectancy of the patient.

In Diabetes Mellitus Type 2, glucose, once absorbed from the intestinal tract and poured into the circulatory stream - due to an alteration of the hormonal vehicle (insulin) or a malfunction of peripheral tyrosine kinase receptors that do not capture it effectively enough - remains in the circulation causing a series of negative metabolic reactions (NB. The nervous tissue is the only insulin-independent).

Diabetes Mellitus Type 2 is a disorder that includes many facets, but what is common to ALL clinical pictures is a situation of hyperglycemia (>110 mg/dl), possibly accompanied by hyper-insulinemia and hyperlipidemia (VLDL - hypertriglyceridemia); Obviously, this frequently leads to overweight, aggravation of hypertension, glycation of plasma proteins, pro-oxidation of APO-protein B and consequent REDUCTION of the ability to bind to peripheral receptors (LDL hypercholesterolemia), increased risk of atherosclerosis, retinopathy, neuropathy, nephropathy and diabetic foot.

Causes and Treatment

Diabetes Mellitus Type 2 has several etiological causes; the most common are related to lifestyle: poor diet and abuse of carbohydrates, excess of fat mass, lack of muscle mass, sedentariness; others are genetic, such as structural alteration of insulin or peripheral receptors. Certainly, whatever the causes, the most effective therapy for Diabetes Mellitus

Type 2 consists of:

- Reducing overweight/obesity
- Reduction of excess carbohydrates and restoration of nutritional balance
- Motor therapy
- Pharmacological therapy
- Compensation of other dysmetabolisms.

Diet for Diabetes Mellitus Type 2

The diet for Diabetes Mellitus Type 2 is almost always constituted by a low-calorie regimen (for weight loss) and, if not hypoglucidic, that provides the least amount of carbohydrates possible while maintaining a certain nutritional balance; the diet for Diabetes Mellitus Type 2 CANNOT be separated from the beginning of a motor therapy.

The basic principles of the diet for Diabetes Mellitus Type 2 are:

- Hypocaloricity (if necessary)
- Reduction of the overall glycemic load
- Reduction of the glycemic load of meals
- Reduction of the glycemic index of meals

Simple carbohydrate intake exclusively represented by fructose naturally present in vegetables or lactose naturally present in milk and dairy products (if possible, simple CHOs should remain around 10-12% of total calories).

Which, from a practical standpoint, translates into:

- Choosing fibre-rich foods and drastically eliminating/reducing refined foods
- Abolition of sweets, sweet carbonated drinks, fruit juices, beer and baked goods
- Reduction of fruit that is too sweet and elimination of preserved fruit (candied, syrupy, jams (questionable), dehydrated etc.)
- Increase, as much as possible, foods containing antioxidants (vegetables, fruits NOT too sugary).

Useful supplements

There are no fundamental supplements to the treatment/diet for Diabetes Mellitus Type 2 (drugs are NOT supplements); however, it is obvious that a well-considered supplementation based on antioxidants (to try to improve the oxidative stress on lipoproteins) and, in the case of a strongly hypocaloric diet, a supplement of fibre (possibly viscous that improve the glycemic index of the meal and increase the sense of satiety) could be useful in improving the impact of nutritional treatment.

Chapter 2 – Recipes for Diabetics and Standards for a Healthy Diet

General Dietary Recommendations

- Reduce consumption of simple sugars.
- Reduce consumption of saturated fats.
- Increase fiber consumption.
- Never skip breakfast.
- Eat complete meals (carbohydrates + protein + vegetables + fruit) at lunch and dinner.
- Avoid prolonged periods of fasting.
- Share equally, in the 3 main meals, the total amount of complex carbohydrates (bread, pasta, rice, rusks).

In following the indications it should be however considered that, in order to obtain a correct and balanced nutrition which supplies the body with all the nutrients it needs, it is necessary to assume the right quantity (portion) of food and to respect the frequency with which some foods must be consumed, daily or weekly, within a personalized food scheme.

The daily nutrition must respect the energy balance of each person and the energy introduced must be equal to the one spent in order not to increase the risk of overweight, obesity as well as malnutrition.

Food not allowed

- White sugar and brown sugar or fructose to sweeten beverages, substituting sweetener if necessary.
- Jam and honey.
- Sweets such as cakes, pastries, cookies, shortbread, jellies, puddings, candies.
- Fruit in syrup, candied fruit, fruit mustard.
- Sugary drinks such as cola, tonic water, iced tea, as well as fruit juices, because they naturally contain sugar even if they are labelled "no added sugar".
- Sauces containing sugar such as ketchup.
- Fatty condiments such as butter, lard, margarine.
- Sausages.
- Spirits.

Food allowed in moderation

It is important to respect the quantities indicated in the diet and limit to occasional consumption the sugariness fruits (grapes, bananas, figs, persimmons, tangerines).

- Fruits as they naturally contain sugar (fructose).
- Sweetener.
- Dietary bakery products for diabetics, remembering that although sugar-free they are not low-calorie, but have a caloric value almost equal to traditional analogues.
- Red wine (about half glass per meal).
- Salt. It is a good rule to reduce the amount of salt added to food during and after cooking and to limit the consumption of foods which naturally contain high quantities of salt (canned or pickled foods, meat cubes and extracts, soy sauces).

- Chestnuts are not a fruit and potatoes and corn are not a vegetable.

These foods are important sources of starch therefore they are real substitutes of bread, pasta and rice.

Therefore they can be occasionally consumed as a substitute of the first course.

- Legumes (chickpeas, beans, peas, broad beans, etc.) should be limited, as they contain carbohydrates and therefore raise blood sugar; however they are also an important source of vegetable proteins (therefore they can be considered as real and proper second courses).

It is advisable to consume them in association with cereals (1 or 2 times a week) therefore making unique dishes.

Allowed and recommended foods

- Raw and cooked vegetables to be consumed in generous portions.
- Fish (fresh or frozen) no less than two to three times a week.
- Complex carbohydrates (bread, pasta, rice, toast) and whole grains.
- Olive oil, added raw and in moderation.
- Cheese to be consumed a couple of times a week, as an alternative to the second course.

- You can take a couple of teaspoons (15 gr) of grated Grana Padano D.O.P. per day.
- Leaner sliced meats (cooked ham, raw ham, bresaola, speck, roast turkey and chicken) depriving them of visible fat.
- Red and white meat (from lean cuts and without visible fat). Skinless poultry.
- Skimmed or semi-skimmed milk and yogurt.
- Water, at least 1.5 litres per day (preferably low-mineral water).

Behavioral Rules

In case of overweight or obesity it is recommended the reduction of weight and of the "waistline", that is the abdominal circumference, indicator of the amount of fat deposited at visceral level.

Waist circumference values above 94 cm in men and 80 cm in women are associated with a "moderate" cardiovascular risk, values above 102 cm in men and 88 cm in women are associated with a "high risk". Returning to a normal weight allows not only to reduce blood glucose levels, but also to reduce other cardiovascular risk factors (such as hypertension, hypercholesterolemia, hypertriglyceridemia).

- Make your lifestyle more active (give up being sedentary! Walk, bike, or park far to work; if you can, avoid using the elevator and walk the stairs).

- Practice physical activity at least three times a week both aerobic and muscle strengthening (anaerobic).

Constant physical activity has beneficial effects on people with diabetes, as well as being essential to eliminate excess fat and lose weight properly.

Read product labels, especially to ascertain their sugar content. Pay attention to the use of "sugar-free" products as they are often rich in fat and consequently high in calories.

Practical Tips

The patient with diabetes mellitus type 2 should include in his diet

- a breakfast consisting of: a cup of semi-skimmed milk or a pot of low-fat yogurt + rusks or bread or cereals or dry cookies plus a medium-sized fruit (about 150 g), to be eaten preferably with the skin, well washed.
- at lunch and dinner complete meals, consisting of: bread, pasta or rice (preferably cooked "al dente", using in about 50% of cases whole grains) plus main course (meat or fish or cheese or sliced meats or eggs or legumes) plus vegetables plus a fruit. Those who do not want to eat first and second course, can make unique dishes based on carbohydrates and proteins such as pasta with tuna, rice and pasta with legumes, pasta with mozzarella and tomato, roast beef sandwich, always accompanied by vegetables and a fruit.

- possible snacks between meals or in the late evening, if you are accustomed to eat dinner early (before 20), based on fresh fruit, low-fat yogurt with a tablespoon of cereals without sugar, or a glass of milk or a few flakes of Parmigiano cheese (10-15 g) with a couple of rusks.

Warnings

The dietary advices provided are purely indicative and must not be considered a substitute for the indications of the doctor, as some patients may require dietary adaptations based on their individual clinical situation.

The ideal diet is one that prefers legumes, fruits, vegetables and whole grains.

Legumes

One of the foods that should never be missing on the table of those who suffer from diabetes (but not only), are legumes. It is, in fact, a super food able to bring numerous benefits to our body.

Legumes, thanks to the high content of soluble fibre, help to keep under control the levels of glucose in the blood.

So, bringing lentils, peas, chickpeas and beans to the table two-three times a week is, without a doubt, a healthy choice. In addition, always the presence of fibre increases the sense of satiety.

All this helps to avoid hunger attacks and various binges responsible for weight gain.

Fruits and vegetables should never be missing in a varied and balanced diet.

Vegetables also play an important role in the diet of diabetics as they help to control the absorption of sugar in the blood.

The ideal is to consume five portions of vegetables a day, varying as much as possible "color" and type.

As for vegetables, they should never be missing in every meal (both at lunch and dinner).

Fruits and vegetables are beneficial for those who suffer from diabetes. Fibre keeps glucose values under control, increases the level of satiety and helps to return to a healthy weight, specifies the expert.

Those who are overweight or obese are more likely to suffer from diabetes.

Whole grain bread and pasta

Who suffers from diabetes should prefer complex carbohydrates, contained in cereals, preferably whole grain.

Green light to pasta or brown rice seasoned with vegetables and legumes, sprinkled with a drizzle of raw evo oil.

First courses based on whole grains, enriched with vegetable sauces, provide an excellent intake of fibre, with beneficial effects on health (glucose and fat under control, greater satiety).

The Mediterranean diet (rich in fruits, vegetables, fish and whole grains) is therefore also suitable for the diet of diabetics.

Not only whole-grain pasta, bread and rice: to vary the diet, you can alternate satisfying pasta dishes to tasty one-dish meals based on cereals and legumes such as, for example, kamut and lentils or, again, couscous of spelt, peas and vegetables.

Attention to drink

Not only food, if you need to keep blood sugar under control you must also pay attention to what you drink.

For example, those who suffer from diabetes should avoid the consumption of sugary drinks, such as: cola, orangeade, sodas, fruit juices and various cocktails.

These are real "sugar bombs" that rapidly raise blood sugar levels.

"In addition, sugary drinks bring the so-called "empty" calories, that is, devoid of nutrition."

Also beware of hidden, well-disguised sugar: contained, for example, in fruit in syrup and sweet snacks.

Prefer foods with low energy density

Among the foods to avoid, to ward off blood sugar spikes, are all those foods with high caloric density.

"Foods that are high in fat and simple sugars but low in water generally provide a lot of energy in a small volume.

These are the energy-dense foods like a slice of chocolate cake or a sandwich with mayonnaise, or even sausages."

Foods rich in water and fibre such as fruits, vegetables and whole grains, on the other hand, provide few calories in a large volume and are defined as low energy density.

The stomach is "deceived" by the volume of food and, therefore, foods or preparations that have a low energy density have a greater satiating power.

An example: first courses based on whole grains, legumes and vegetables.

A glass of wine a day

Alcohol, in case one suffers from diabetes or if one is overweight, should be avoided.

In case, once in a while, one wants to indulge in a glass of wine, it is appropriate to keep an eye on the quantity allowed.

A moderate intake of alcohol, up to 10 grams/day for women (one serving) and 20 grams/day for men (two servings), is acceptable.

However, diabetics should avoid drinks such as hard liquor cocktails altogether.

The same goes for non-alcoholic mixes, which are very rich in simple sugars and empty calories.

Lots of fibre

pasta al dente, cold potatoes: here are the practical suggestions for the diet of those who have problems with insulin.

Strict restrictions in the diet of those with type 2 diabetes, the most common?

That era is gone, because some tricks allow you to eat in a tasty way trying to keep blood sugar at bay. Or by respecting certain dietary regimens or by learning some simple rules to cook in a healthier way.

There are also some clichés to dismantle. Contrary to popular belief, the basis for a balanced diet in diabetics is also carbohydrate and fibre-rich foods such as fruits and vegetables.

Diabetes and hypertension.

In short, the plate of spaghetti is welcome. Today, diabetes is no longer considered, as it was a few years ago, a kind of allergy to sugar.

Carbohydrates are not only allowed, but recommended, because they are necessary for the body.

So how should the diet be for those who have problems with insulin?

I try to summarize a simple message for the choices at the table in type 2 diabetes: you can eat anything, but you can't eat a lot.

A 5-10% weight loss is enough to optimize disease control, but also to halve the risk of becoming diabetic in an overweight or obese person.

The problem is growing.

According to the latest data, Italians with type 2 diabetes (non-autoimmune) are over 3.5 million and in 2030 will be, according to estimates, over 5 million.

This is a chronic disease, characterized by the presence of high levels of glucose in the blood (hyperglycemia) and due to an altered amount or activity of insulin (the hormone, produced by the pancreas, which allows glucose to enter the cells and its subsequent use as an energy source).

To cope with it, you need to change your eating habits.

Throughout life.

But it must be experienced as a change, not as a deprivation.

Often totally eliminating certain foods can be more dangerous than indulging in them in a reasoned way.

Here are some tips on proper nutrition for diabetics.

With one caveat: it is advisable to define a personalized diet plan with a specialist.

Tricks for lowering the glycemic index.

It is useful for a diabetic to learn to distinguish foods based on the glycemic index.

This parameter indicates how quickly the glucose in food is absorbed by the blood.

When we eat a food rich in carbohydrates, glucose levels in the bloodstream gradually increase as starches and sugars are digested and assimilated.

The speed of these processes changes according to the food and the type of nutrients it contains, the amount of fibre present and the composition of other foods already present in the stomach and intestine.

The glycemic index is mainly related to foods high in carbohydrates, whereas those rich in fat or proteins do not have an immediate effect on blood sugar levels (glycemia), but determine a delayed and prolonged increase.

The glycemic index is influenced by the composition of foods, but also by cooking methods.

They tend to reduce it, for example, the partial boiling (spaghetti al dente and not cooked are

good in every sense) or the cooling of cooked foods, such as boiled potatoes.

Also the presence of foods with soluble fibres, capable of absorbing high quantities of water, forming in the intestine a sort of gel, helps to lower the glycemic index.

But what happens, instead, if you overdo with foods with high glycemic index?

A rapid rise in blood sugar levels causes the pancreas to secrete large amounts of insulin.

And insulin causes a rapid utilization of glucose by the tissues, so that two-three hours after the meal, hypoglycemia is determined, resulting in a feeling of hunger and a certain discomfort. If you ingest more carbohydrates to cope with hunger, you stimulate a new secretion of insulin and you enter a vicious circle.

This is not the only danger.

Often the body doesn't use all the glucose, so it is converted into fat tissue.

Unused fat reserves accumulate and generate overweight.

Not all scholars, however, evaluate the usefulness of the glycemic index in the same way.

The American Diabetes Association (ADA) has even questioned its clinical usefulness, recommending that attention be paid more to the quantity of food than to the source of carbohydrates.

A well-balanced diet is the essential cure for diabetes.

First Courses

Bulgur with cream of peppers

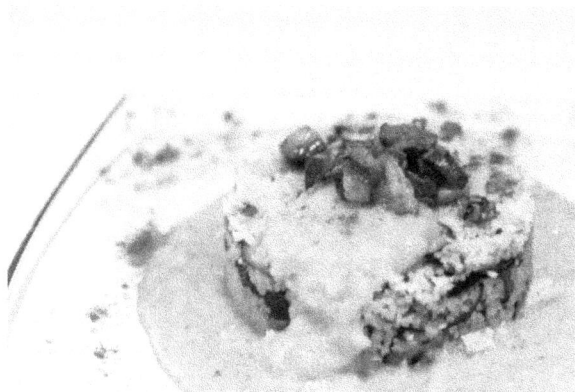

Recipe ID card

~ 78 Kcal calories per serving
~ Difficulty very easy
~ Serves 2
~ Preparation 15 minutes
~ Low cost
~ 15 minutes + time for washing and cutting vegetables

Ingredients

~ 150 g of bulgur
~ 300 ml of water
~ 200 g of zucchini
~ 200 g of eggplants
~ 200 g of peppers
~ 2 tablespoons (20 ml) extra virgin olive oil
~ 1 teaspoon of sweet paprika
~ 1 pinch of salt
~ pepper

Material Required

~ Casserole with lid
~ Stone pans of various sizes
~ Immersion mixer and container
~ Serving dish
~ Knife
~ Chopping board
~ Ladles and spoons
~ Pasta cup for serving (optional)

Preparation

Pour the water into a small saucepan and bring to a boil. Season with salt, turn off the heat and pour in the bulgur. Stir quickly and cover the saucepan with the lid. Let the bulgur rest for 10 minutes, without stirring or lifting the lid: in this way, the bulgur, by absorbing all the water, will swell.

While the bulgur is cooking, prepare the vegetables. Thoroughly wash zucchini and eggplant, remove ends and reduce vegetables into small cubes. Then wash the bell pepper, remove the non-edible parts (including seeds and filaments) and cut it into small pieces.

Put two frying pans on the fire so that they become very hot. In a large pan, pour zucchini and eggplant (which will serve as a sauce for the bulgur), while in the other the peppers (which will then be blended and reduced to a cream). Add a dash of oil and a pinch of salt to each pan and cook for about ten minutes over high heat.

Once the peppers have browned to perfection, lower the heat and let them wilt for another 5 minutes. Transfer the peppers to a beaker and blend with an immersion blender until creamy.

In the meantime, the bulgur will have absorbed all the water: shell it with a spoon or a fork and add it to the sautéed vegetables, with a pinch of sweet paprika.

Pour the bell pepper cream in a serving dish. Place a pasta cup in the center of the sauce, then fill with bulgur. Gently flatten the bulgur with a spoon so that it takes on the shape of the mold.

Remove the noodle dish and serve decorating with a little bell pepper cream, vegetables and a sprinkling of sweet paprika.

Cream of pumpkin and potatoes

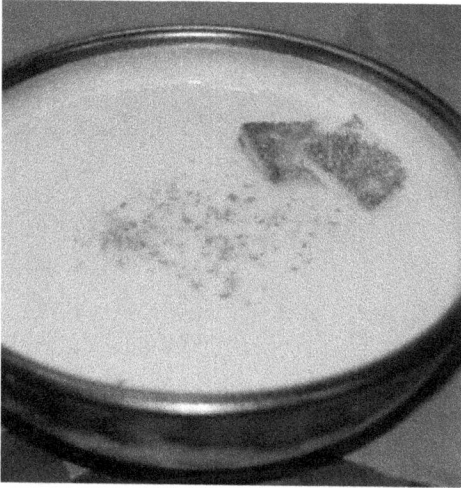

Recipe ID card

- ~ 92 Kcal calories per serving
- ~ Easy difficulty
- ~ Serves 3
- ~ Preparation 26 minutes
- ~ Low cost
- ~ 5-6 minutes to prepare; 15-20 minutes to cook

Ingredients

- ~ 2 glasses (about 400 ml) of water
- ~ 300 ml (a glass and a half) of milk
- ~ 2 tablespoons (30 ml) of extra virgin olive oil
- ~ 5 slices of bread
- ~ 200 g (2 medium-sized) potatoes
- ~ 1 pinch of pepper
- ~ 2 sprigs of rosemary
- ~ salt
- ~ 350 g of pumpkin

Material Required

- ~ 1 food cutting board
- ~ 1 sharp knife to remove the rind from the pumpkin
- ~ 1 spoon for removing seeds from pumpkin
- ~ 1 wooden spoon for stirring the cream
- ~ 1 stone or non-stick pan for cooking the pumpkin puree
- ~ 1 potato peeler to peel the potatoes
- ~ 1 immersion blender
- ~ 1 bread knife
- ~ 1 ladle for serving the pumpkin puree
- ~ 1 serving plate

Preparation

Prepare the pumpkin: first remove the seeds, then the peel, being very careful not to cut with the knife. At this point, cut the pumpkin into small cubes and place them in a small bowl.

Prepare the potatoes. With the help of a potato peeler, peel the vegetables and cut them into small pieces. Combine the potato cubes with the pumpkin cubes.

In the meantime, put on the stove a large pot and, when it will be very hot, brown potatoes and pumpkin, without adding oil, butter or sauté: in this way, it will be possible to taste the real flavor of vegetables.

After pumpkin and potatoes begin to form a light golden crust, add the equivalent of 2 glasses of water in the pot of vegetables.

Season with salt and pepper, stir quickly and bring to a boil. Close the pot with the lid and cook, stirring occasionally, for about 15-20 minutes, until the vegetables have reached a fairly creamy consistency.

In the meantime, prepare the croutons that will be used to top the cream of pumpkin and potato soup. Remove the edge from 5 slices of bread with a knife; cut out many small cubes. Put a large frying pan on the stove and, when hot, add two tablespoons of oil and a sprig of rosemary; then, pour the bread cubes and let them brown well. If necessary, add a little salt to make the croutons tastier.

After 20 minutes, the vegetables will have reached a creamy consistency. At this point, with the help of an immersion blender, make the vegetables into a cream. To facilitate the operation, gradually add 1 ½ glasses of milk, possibly hot. In order to flavor the soup, add a sprig of rosemary to the obtained cream and leave it in the soup until the moment of serving. For a more delicate taste, add the rosemary after having removed the soup from the heat.

The soup should be served hot, accompanied by a handful of croutons and a sprig of rosemary in order to make the presentation even more pleasing.

Strawberry Gazpacho

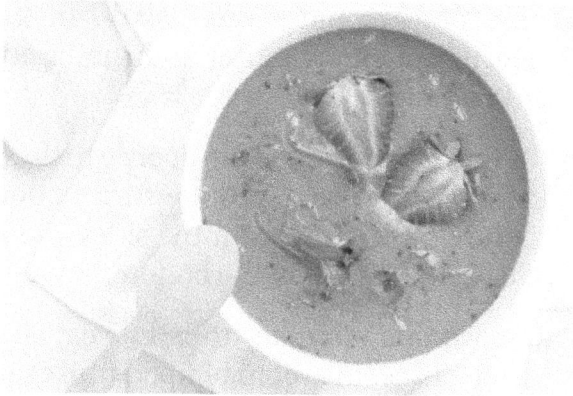

Preparation

Clean the strawberries: remove the stems, wash them in cold water and gently dry them with paper towels.

Cut the strawberries into pieces and pour them into the glass of the blender.

Wash the cucumber, peel it and cut it into pieces. Add the cucumber to the strawberries.

Add the peeled tomatoes, ginger (powdered or fresh), coriander seeds and mint leaves.

Season with salt and pepper to taste, then add a dash of balsamic vinegar glaze (or just balsamic vinegar). Add a few ice cubes and blend everything together.

Distribute the resulting gazpacho in individual glasses and garnish with mint leaves and strawberry slices.

Recipe ID card

~ 52 Kcal calories per serving
~ Easy difficulty
~ Serves 4
~ Preparation 15 minutes
~ Low cost

Ingredients

~ 100 g of cucumbers
~ salt
~ 200 g of tomato puree or coppery tomatoes
~ pepper
~ A few mint leaves
~ A splash of balsamic vinegar glaze
~ A few ice cubes
~ 300 g of strawberries
~ 1 tablespoon of coriander seeds
~ 1 piece of fresh ginger or 1 teaspoon of ginger powder

Material Required

~ Glass blender
~ Vegetable peeler
~ Glasses
~ Chopping board

Parisian style gnocchi

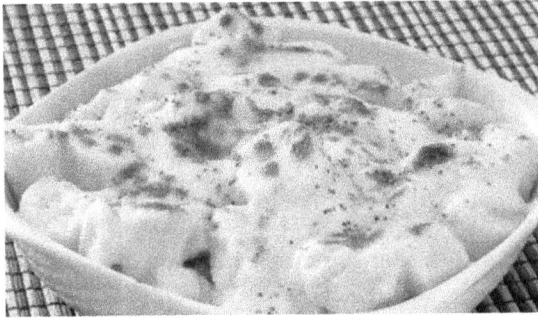

Recipe ID card

- ~ 185 Kcal calories per serving
- ~ Difficulty fairly easy
- ~ Serves 3
- ~ Preparation 30 minutes
- ~ Low cost
- ~ 30 minutes + time for au gratin in the oven

Ingredients

For the dough

- ~ 125 ml of milk
- ~ 60 g of butter
- ~ 1 pinch of salt
- ~ 75 g of white flour type 00
- ~ 120 g (2 medium-sized) eggs
- ~ 1 grated nutmeg

For the dressing and gratin

- ~ 250 g of light béchamel sauce
- ~ about 30 g of grated Parmesan cheese

Material Required

- ~ Saucepan
- ~ Large saucepan
- ~ Whisk
- ~ Precision scales
- ~ Wooden spoon
- ~ Sac à poche
- ~ Pyrex dish
- ~ Knife
- ~ Skimmer

Preparation

First, prepare the choux pastry. In a small saucepan, melt the butter in the milk, add salt and nutmeg.

Sift the flour and add it all at once to the butter and milk mixture. Continue stirring until the mixture pulls away from the sides and a thin layer of foil forms on the bottom.

Remove the saucepan from the heat and add, one at a time, the room temperature eggs. It is recommended not to add the second egg if the first one has not been completely absorbed by the mixture.

Prepare the béchamel sauce without butter. Spread some of the béchamel in the bottom of a large Pyrex dish.

Meanwhile, boil a saucepan with plenty of lightly salted water. Transfer the choux pastry mixture to a piping bag with a smooth nozzle.

As soon as the water begins to boil, place the sac à poche over the casserole and push the mixture to the end of the pocket: obtain small dumplings with the help of a knife. We recommend referring to the video. Using a skimmer, gradually remove the gnocchi from the cooking water as soon as they begin to float, and place them in the oven dish with the béchamel sauce. Continue in this way until all the dough is used up.

Cover the gnocchi with the remaining béchamel sauce, sprinkle with grated Parmesan cheese and bake at 180°C for 15 minutes or in the microwave for 5 minutes (combined micro-grill function).

Serve the gnocchi steaming hot.

Barley with zucchini and saffron

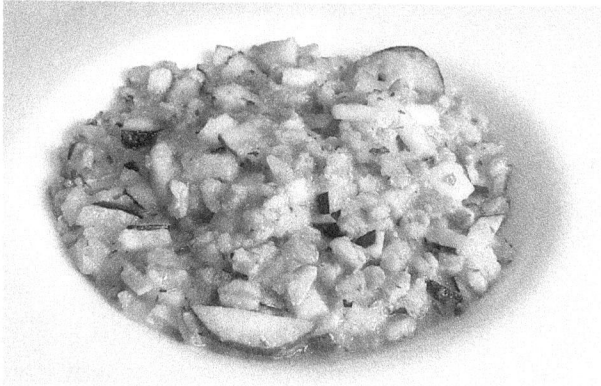

Recipe ID card

~ 103 Kcal calories per serving
~ Easy difficulty
~ Serves 2
~ Preparation 30 minutes
~ Low cost
~ 30 minutes + time to prepare vegetable stock

Ingredients

~ about half a litre of vegetable broth
~ 1 or 2 tablespoons (10 or 20 ml) of extra-virgin olive oil
~ 150 g of pearl barley
~ of pepper
~ 1 tuft of parsley
~ a pinch of salt
~ 1 sachet of saffron
~ 200 g of zucchini

Material Required

~ Pot for vegetable stock
~ Casserole for preparing the barley
~ Pan for browning zucchini
~ Becker + immersion blender for the cream of zucchini
~ Chopping board and knives for preparing the zucchini
~ Wooden and steel ladles

Preparation

Prepare the vegetable broth by boiling half a litre of salted water with a carrot, a zucchini and a potato (alternatively, you can use vegetable stock cube or powder).

Clean and wash the zucchini thoroughly, removing the non-edible parts. Cut the zucchini into small pieces and brown them in a pan with a little extra-virgin olive oil, salt and pepper.

When the zucchini are browned on all sides (2-3 minutes will be enough), pour part of it into a casserole: add the barley and let it toast for a few minutes. The remaining zucchini will be creamed later.

At this point, proceed as you would a normal risotto, gradually hydrating the barley with a little hot broth at a time. The optimal cooking time for pearl barley is 30 minutes.

After 20 minutes, the remaining zucchini (which have finished cooking in the pan) will have become soft: pour them into a beaker and reduce them to a cream with the immersion blender, adding a little hot broth if necessary.

Add the cream of zucchini in the pot of barley. Dissolve the saffron in a little stock, then add it to the barley.

Continue stirring to distribute the saffron and the cream of zucchini well. Finish cooking, seasoning with a little fresh parsley.

Arrange a few slices of grilled zucchini on a plate (optional) and serve immediately decorating with a leaf of parsley and zucchini curls.

Vegetarian Paella

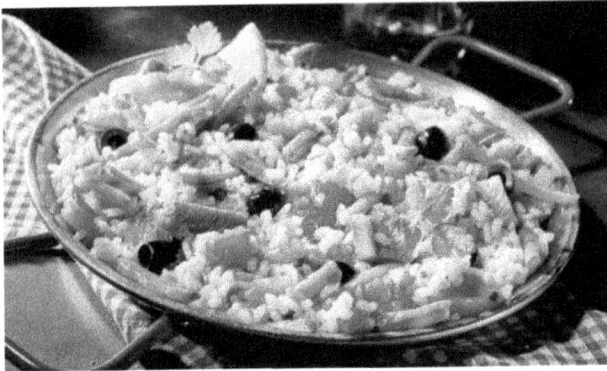

Recipe ID card

- ~ 89 Kcal calories per serving
- ~ Difficulty fairly easy
- ~ Serves 4
- ~ Preparation 40 minutes
- ~ Average cost

Ingredients

- ~ 300 g of brown rice
- ~ salt
- ~ 3 tablespoons (about 30 ml) of extra virgin olive oil
- ~ 1 sachet of saffron
- ~ Home-made food: 30 g of vegetable stock cube
- ~ A few basil leaves
- ~ 1 tuft of parsley
- ~ 150 g of peppers
- ~ 150 g of seitan
- ~ 150 g of carrots
- ~ 150 g of zucchini
- ~ 150 g of cherry tomatoes
- ~ Shelled, fresh food: 150 g of broad beans
- ~ about 750-780 ml of water
- ~ pepper

Material Required

- ~ Paella pan
- ~ Cutting board
- ~ Lid
- ~ Spoon
- ~ Casserole

Preparation

Bring water to a boil and season with a tablespoon of homemade cream vegetable stock cube.

Meanwhile, wash all the vegetables. Shell the broad beans, cut the bell pepper into strips (after removing the seeds and internal filaments), dice the zucchini and carrots and cherry tomatoes into small pieces.

Heat three tablespoons of oil in a large saucepan, then combine all the vegetables, except for the broad beans, adding salt and pepper to taste. Sauté the vegetables over high heat for 5 minutes.

Sauté the diced seitan and season with salt and pepper.

Rinse the brown parboiled rice and add it to the vegetables. Add the broad beans and mix thoroughly.

Pour in the water, cover with the lid and cook, avoiding stirring, for about 15-20 minutes.

Five minutes before the rice is cooked, dissolve a sachet of saffron in a tablespoon of hot water and add it to the rice.

Turn off heat and finish with aromatic herbs as desired, such as parsley and basil.

Pasta with Fresh Tuna

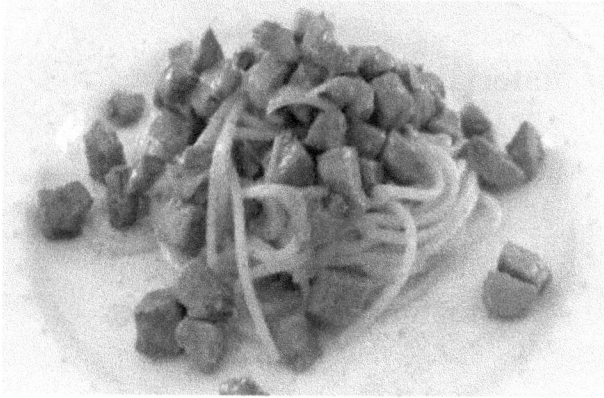

Recipe ID card

- ~ 158 Kcal calories per serving
- ~ Easy difficulty
- ~ Serves 4
- ~ Preparation 20 minutes
- ~ Average cost

Ingredients

- ~ 320 g of whole wheat spaghetti or another type of whole wheat pasta
- ~ 250 g of fresh tuna
- ~ 30 g of capers
- ~ 400 g of canned cherry tomatoes
- ~ 1 sprig of parsley
- ~ 2 tablespoons (about 20 ml) of extra virgin olive oil
- ~ salt
- ~ 1 clove of garlic
- ~ Half a small glass of brandy

Material Required

- ~ Cutting board
- ~ Knife
- ~ Sauce casserole
- ~ Casserole for pasta
- ~ Frying pan
- ~ Pasta strainer
- ~ Spaghetti fork

Preparation

Prepare the tomato sauce. In a saucepan, bring together the canned tomatoes (or fresh tomatoes), a clove of garlic, the salt and capers. Cover with the lid and let cook slowly for 15 minutes, stirring occasionally.

Meanwhile, cut the fresh tuna into thin slices.

Heat a frying pan and add 2 tablespoons of e.v.o. oil. When the oil is hot, fry the fresh tuna over high heat for 2-3 minutes. Deglaze the tuna with brandy or half a small glass of dry white wine: allow the alcohol to evaporate, stirring frequently for about a minute. Turn off the heat: tuna does not require a long cooking time.

Bring plenty of water to the boil and add salt to taste. When water boils, add whole-wheat spaghetti (or another type of whole-wheat pasta): for cooking times, check package.

A few minutes before the end of cooking the pasta, add the browned tuna to the tomato sauce and remove the garlic. If the sauce is excessively dry, add one or two tablespoons of pasta water. Taste for flavor and, if necessary, add a pinch of salt.

Drain the pasta and toss with the sauce. Turn off the flame and flavor with fresh parsley.

Pasta and Beans

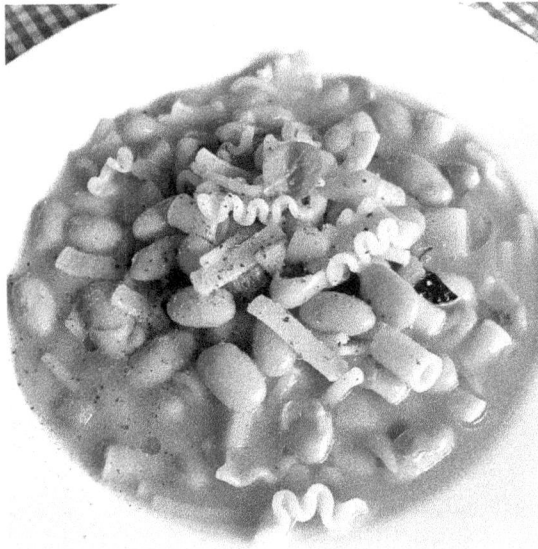

~ 1 celery stalk

Material Required

- ~ Bowls
- ~ Pastry board
- ~ Wooden spoon
- ~ Pasta machine or rolling pin
- ~ Knife or pasta cutter wheel
- ~ Large saucepan
- ~ Scoop
- ~ Frying pan with lid
- ~ Vegetable mixer

Preparation

Rinse beans from soaking water to remove anti-nutritional substances. Plunge them into a saucepan filled with cold water and bring to a boil: cook for 1 hour and a half or two. It is recommended to add salt at the end: salt in fact tends to harden the outer coating.

In the meantime, prepare the accompanying sauce. Wash carrot and celery thoroughly. Peel the carrot and remove any filaments from the celery. Cut the vegetables into small pieces and finely chop them in a blender.

Brown the vegetables in a saucepan, adding a drizzle of oil and a little salt. Add the peeled tomatoes and continue cooking for 10 minutes.

Prepare the pasta. Make maltagliati with the help of a knife or pasta cutter.

Remove the boiled beans from the cooking broth, using a skimmer. Sauté the beans in the sauce, adding a couple of ladles of the broth.

Dip the fresh pasta directly into the sauce and continue cooking for 5-7 minutes.

Finish cooking by adding a sprig of rosemary to the pasta.

Recipe ID card

- ~ 115 Kcal calories per serving
- ~ Difficulty fairly easy
- ~ Serves 4
- ~ Preparation 120 minutes
- ~ Low cost
- ~ 2 for preparation of the dish + soaking time of beans (1 night)

Ingredients

For the fresh pasta (maltagliati)

- ~ 100 g of white flour type 00
- ~ 100 g of remilled durum wheat semolina
- ~ 120 g (2 medium) eggs

For the sauce

- ~ 1 pinch of salt
- ~ 1 sprig of rosemary
- ~ 100 g of peeled or canned tomatoes
- ~ 1 sprinkling of pepper
- ~ 2 tablespoons of extra virgin olive oil
- ~ 200 g of dried beans
- ~ 150 g of carrots
- ~ water

Wholewheat pasta with peppers

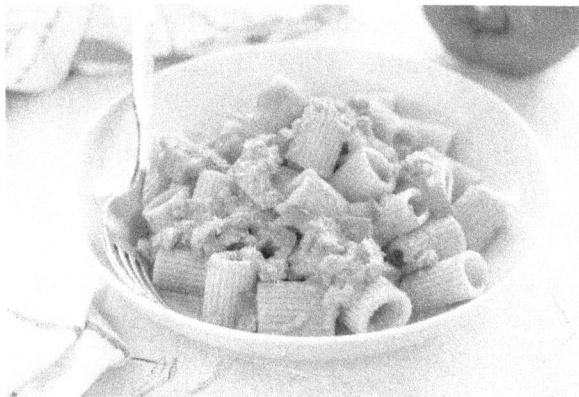

Recipe ID card

~ 122 Kcal calories per serving
~ Easy difficulty
~ Serves 2
~ Preparation 15 minutes
~ Low cost
~ 15 minutes + time to prepare fresh whole wheat pasta

Ingredients

~ 120 g of fresh whole wheat pasta
~ 400 g of peppers
~ 2 tablespoons of extra virgin olive oil
~ 1 pinch of salt
~ pepper
~ 1 teaspoon of sweet paprika
~ 30 g of grated Parmesan cheese
~ 1 sprig of parsley

Material Required

~ Frying pan
~ Large saucepan with lid
~ Food cutter
~ Knife preferably ceramic
~ Wooden spoon
~ Grater

Preparation

Clean the peppers: wash them in cold water, cut them in half and remove the stalk, filaments and internal seeds. Cut cleaned peppers into matchsticks.

To increase the digestibility of peppers, it is advisable to let them soak in a solution of cold water and salt for at least 20 minutes.

Drain the peppers from the soaking water, rinse them under running water and sauté them in a pan with a little oil, salt, pepper and sweet paprika. Continue cooking for about ten minutes.

In the meantime, bring the water to a boil, add salt to taste and add the fresh whole-wheat pasta. Cook for 5 minutes or more, depending on the thickness of the pasta. If necessary, pour a dash of oil into the cooking water to prevent the pasta from sticking.

Before the pasta is done cooking, remove it from the water with a skimmer and finish cooking in the pan of bell pepper sauce.

Finally, add the chopped parsley and serve with a generous grating of parmesan cheese.

Serve the pasta steaming hot.

Fresh Homemade Wholemeal Pasta

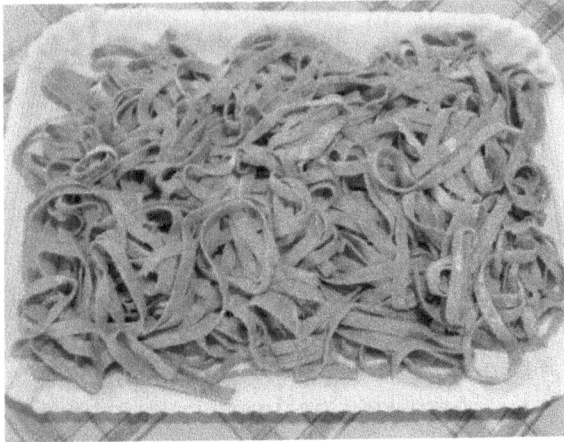

Recipe ID card

~ 244 Kcal calories per serving
~ Difficulty fairly easy
~ Serves 4
~ Preparation 15 minutes
~ Low cost
~ 15 minutes + cooking time

Ingredients

~ 180 g of wholemeal flour
~ 20 g of oat bran
~ 40 g of remilled durum wheat semolina
~ 60 g (1 medium) of eggs
~ 70 ml of water

Material Required

~ Bowl
~ Flattener
~ Precision scales
~ Latex gloves (optional)
~ Rolling pin or pasta machine
~ Pasta cutter wheel
~ Transparent film

Preparation

In a large bowl, mix all the dry ingredients, namely whole wheat flour, remilled durum wheat semolina and oat bran.

Shell an egg and add it to the flour mix along with the water. Knead thoroughly and for a long time, first in the bowl and then on the pastry board: the dough should be compact, smooth but not too firm. If necessary, add more whole wheat flour.

Wrap the dough in a sheet of plastic wrap in order to avoid the formation of a superficial crust, then let the dough rest for 30 minutes. Resting is important in order to make it easier to roll out the dough.

Roll out the dough with a rolling pin or with the proper pasta machine, until a sheet of dough not too thin is obtained. Pasta can be cut at will: spaghetti, lasagnette, taglierini, pappardelle, farfalle etc..

Wholewheat Pasta with Courgette and Ricotta Sauce

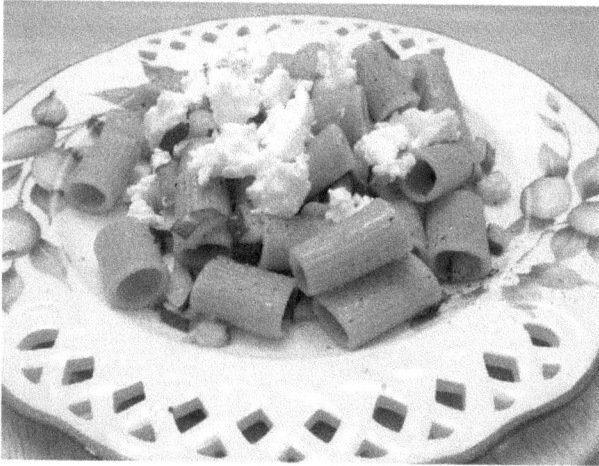

Recipe ID card

- 121 Kcal calories per serving
- Difficulty very easy
- Serves 4
- Preparation 20 minutes
- Low cost
- 15 minutes for preparing pasta and sauce + 5 minutes for cooking

Ingredients

For the dough

- 120 g (2 medium) eggs
- 100 g of remilled durum wheat semolina
- 100 g of whole wheat flour
- 20 g of inulin
- 10 g of soy lecithin

For the seasoning

- salt
- 2 tablespoons (20 ml) of extra virgin olive oil
- 30 g of grated Parmesan cheese
- 1 sprig of parsley
- 125 g of fresh ricotta cheese
- 400 g of zucchinis
- pepe

Material Required

- Large bowl
- Wooden spoon
- Pasta machine or rolling pin
- Pasta cutter or knife
- Latex gloves (optional)
- Pastry board
- Casserole for boiling pasta
- Pan for sauce
- Cheese grater

Preparation

Wash zucchini and remove ends. Cut zucchini lengthwise, until long matchsticks are obtained.

Brown the zucchini in a frying pan, adding a couple of tablespoons of extra virgin olive oil. Season with salt and pepper to taste.

While the sauce is cooking, prepare the pasta. Pour all the dry ingredients, namely the remilled durum wheat semolina, whole wheat flour, inulin and soy lecithin, into a bowl. Mix with your hands or a wooden spoon to blend the powders.

Add two whole eggs and mix vigorously until all the flour is absorbed. If necessary, add more semolina: the dough should not be sticky nor too hard.

Knead the dough for a long time, by hand, until a very elastic and smooth dough is obtained.

Roll out the dough with an electric pasta machine until you obtain sheets 3-4 mm thick. Cut out lasagnette or pappardelle.

Flour the pasta well with semolina to prevent the lasagnette from sticking together.

Plunge the lasagnette into lightly salted boiling water and, if necessary, add a drop of oil directly into the saucepan to prevent the pasta from sticking.

Drain the pasta al dente (a few minutes will be enough, depending on the thickness of the lasagnette) and season with the zucchini sauce.

Finish with a few clumps of fresh ricotta and a generous handful of fresh parsley. Serve with a sprinkling of grated parmesan cheese.

Protein Pasta with Verdure

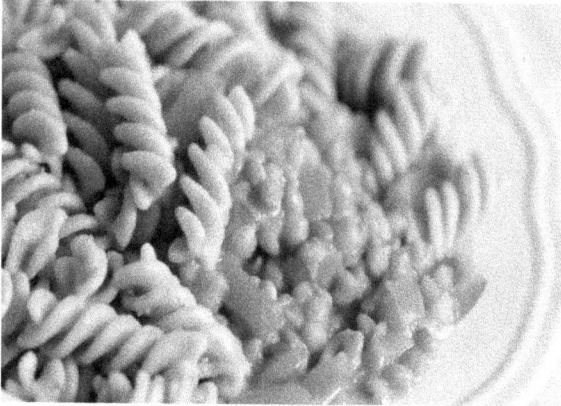

Recipe ID card

- ~ 154 Kcal calories per serving
- ~ Difficulty fairly easy
- ~ Serves 4
- ~ Preparation 25 minutes
- ~ Average cost
- ~ 15 minutes to prepare + 10 minutes to cook

Ingredients

For the pasta

- ~ 110 g of remilled durum wheat semolina
- ~ 25 ml of water
- ~ 40 g (1 medium) egg white
- ~ 60 g (1 whole) of egg
- ~ 7 g of inulin
- ~ 10 g of soy lecithin
- ~ 30 g of whey protein
- ~ 110 g of white flour type 00

For the sauce

- ~ 150 g of carrots
- ~ 250 g of zucchini
- ~ 2 tablespoons of extra virgin olive oil
- ~ salt
- ~ pepper

Material Required

- ~ Rolling pin or electric machine for rolling out the dough
- ~ Sieve for sifting flour
- ~ Pot for cooking pasta
- ~ Pan for cooking vegetables
- ~ Wooden spoon
- ~ 1 ladle (skimmer)
- ~ 1 tray to store the pasta (optional)
- ~ Cloth or plastic wrap to cover the pasta
- ~ 1 zigzag pasta cutter wheel

Preparation

Prepare the vegetarian sauce for the pasta. After washing and cleaning the vegetables, julienne chop both carrots and zucchini using the appropriate machine.

Pour 2 tablespoons of oil into a large skillet and sauté the vegetables over high heat for 5 minutes, adding salt and pepper to taste. Then lower the heat, cover the pan with a lid and continue cooking slowly, stirring occasionally.

In the meantime, prepare the pasta: in a bowl, combine the sifted flour, semolina, inulin, soy lecithin and ultra-microfiltered whey protein. Mix well with a wooden spoon.

Then add the egg whites, the whole egg and the water and mix all the ingredients well.

At this point, divide the dough into two parts: wrap the first ball in a sheet of plastic wrap, to prevent the surface from drying out. Roll out the remaining dough with a rolling pin or with an electric machine. To avoid breaking the dough, it is advisable to roll out the dough to a thickness of at least 3 mm.

After rolling out the dough sheet, cut out many small rectangles of the approximate size of 3x2 cm. With thumb and forefinger of one hand, close each rectangle of dough in the center forming a bow. The dough must not be too dry (be careful not to overdo the flour!) otherwise the edges of the rectangle do not adhere and the butterfly does not form.

Proceed in this manner until the pasta is used up.

In the meantime, the vegetable sauce will be ready.

Plunge the pasta into plenty of boiling salted water and cook for 5-6 minutes. When cooked, transfer the farfalle to the sauce and sauté for one minute.

Vegetarian whole wheat crepes pie

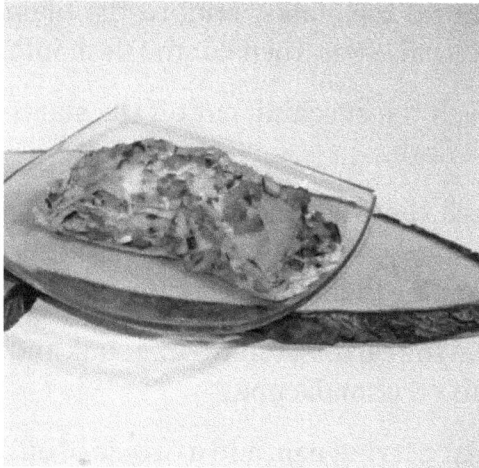

Recipe ID card

- ~ 127 Kcal calories per serving
- ~ Difficulty fairly easy
- ~ Serves 4
- ~ Preparation 45 minutes
- ~ Average cost
- ~ 5 minutes to prepare dough; 15 minutes for crepes; 25 minutes to bake in oven

Ingredients

For the crespelle

- ~ 100 g of white flour type 00
- ~ 50 g of wholemeal flour
- ~ 20 g of butter
- ~ 180 g (3 medium-sized) eggs
- ~ 500 ml of milk
- ~ salt

For the filling

- ~ salt
- ~ 1 tablespoon (10 ml) extra virgin olive oil
- ~ 200 g of Fontina cheese
- ~ 200 g (flesh) of pumpkin
- ~ 400 g (4 large) zucchini
- ~ pepper

Material Required

- ~ 1 whisk (or 1 electric mixer)
- ~ 1 classic or crepe ladle
- ~ 1 non-stick scoop for turning the crepes
- ~ 1 hinged baking pan 26 cm in diameter
- ~ 1 pan for cooking vegetables
- ~ 1 pan for cooking crepes
- ~ baking paper
- ~ 1 knife
- ~ 1 cutting board for food

Preparation

First, make the crepes by mixing the two types of flour, eggs, milk, melted butter and salt until a liquid, smooth, lump-free batter is obtained.

In a hot stone frying pan pour a small ladleful of batter; flip the pancake several times until the surface appears lightly browned. Cook each crepe for a couple of minutes, until all the batter is used up.

In the meantime, prepare the filling for the crepes: cut 200 g of pumpkin pulp and 400 g of zucchini into small squares. Fry the diced mixture in a pan greased with a little oil, season with salt and pepper to taste, and cook until the vegetables are cooked and begin to form a thick cream (about 15 minutes).

In the meantime, blend the string cheese (e.g. fontina), and prepare it on a small bowl.

Prepare a hinged baking dish (diameter 26) and line it with baking paper. Place each crespella in the dish and cover it with a generous amount of vegetables; then proceed by placing a spoonful of grated pasta filata cheese. Cover again with another crespella, the filling and the cheese; proceed in this way until all the ingredients have been used up.

Finish the surface of the pie by sprinkling with a little cheese. Bake in a hot oven at 180°C for 25-30 minutes.

Rice 5 Calories

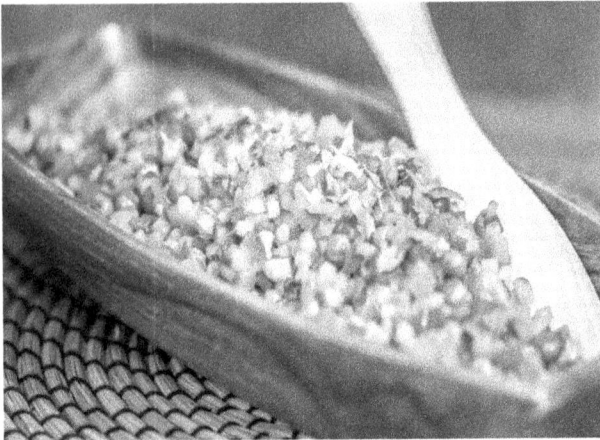

Recipe ID card

~ 42 Kcal calories per serving
~ Easy difficulty
~ Serves 2
~ Preparation 30 minutes
~ Low cost

Ingredients

~ 250 g of konjac gum rice
~ 1 teaspoon of sweet paprika
~ pepper
~ salt
~ 2 tablespoons of extra virgin olive oil
~ 120 g of peas
~ 120 g of zucchini
~ 120 g of carrots
~ 120 g of peppers
~ 1 tuft of parsley

Material Required

~ Colander
~ Saucepan with lid
~ Cutting board
~ Knife
~ Frying pan with lid

Preparation

Clean the vegetables. Wash the peppers, remove the stalks, remove the filaments and internal seeds, then cut the flesh into strips.

Wash the zucchini, cut off the stalks and dice the flesh.

Shell the peas and boil them in water for 10 minutes. Alternatively, defrost the peas and combine them with the remaining vegetables.

Peel the carrots, remove the stalk and cut them into very small cubes.

Heat a frying pan, add a drizzle of oil and sauté the vegetables (carrots, zucchini, peppers and peas) while maintaining a medium-high flame. Adjust salt and pepper, flavouring to taste with sweet paprika. After the vegetables have browned, lower the heat, cover with the lid and cook for 10 minutes.

Meanwhile, fill a small pot with water and bring to a boil.

Open the package of konjac rice and rinse it in cold running water.

Plunge the rice into the boiling water and cook for 2 minutes.

Drain the rice and add it to the vegetables.

Let it season for a couple of minutes and serve immediately with fresh parsley.

Gently roll up the pastry, trying to fold in the ends: this will prevent the filling from escaping during cooking.

Close the roll like a candy, using a kitchen string. Gently plunge the roll of dough into lightly salted water and simmer for about 45 minutes.

Meanwhile, prepare the accompanying tomato sauce. In a small saucepan, pour in the tomato puree, add a drizzle of oil, salt and pepper, and let everything season for 10-15 minutes. Those who wish can add a few basil leaves or a clove of garlic.

When the roll of pasta is proto, remove it from the cooking water, let it drain and remove it from the dish towel. The roll is ready to be cut into slices.

Serve the roll slices accompanied by the tomato sauce. Those who wish can sprinkle with a little grated grana cheese.

Konjac shirataki

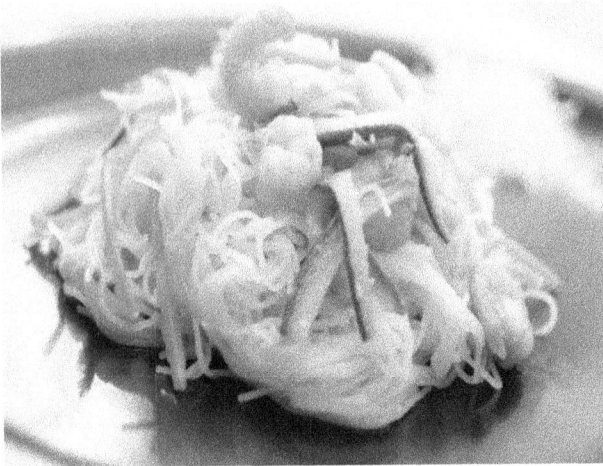

Recipe ID card

~ 47 Kcal calories per serving
~ Difficulty very easy
~ Serves 2
~ Preparation 15 minutes
~ Low cost

Ingredients

~ 250 g of konjac noodles
~ 200 g of peppers
~ 100 g of cherry tomatoes
~ soy sauce
~ 1 sprig of parsley
~ 2 tablespoons of sunflower oil or corn seed oil
~ 1 pinch of salt

Material Required

~ Colander
~ Frying pan
~ Cutting board
~ Knives

Preparation

Clean the peppers: wash the vegetables under running water, removing the stem, seeds and internal filaments. Cut the peppers into very thin slices.

Pour two tablespoons of oil into a frying pan and brown the peppers for a few minutes, turning them often. Flavor with soy sauce and add pepper to taste.

Cook for 5 minutes, or until peppers are soft in texture.

Open package of konjac shirataki noodles, rinse in cold water.

Bring a small pot of lightly salted water to a boil and plunge the noodles in. Let them heat for a couple of minutes, then drain and toss them in the bell pepper sauce.

Serve the konjac shirataki spaghetti with plenty of freshly chopped parsley.

Whole wheat spaghetti with cream, lemon and walnuts

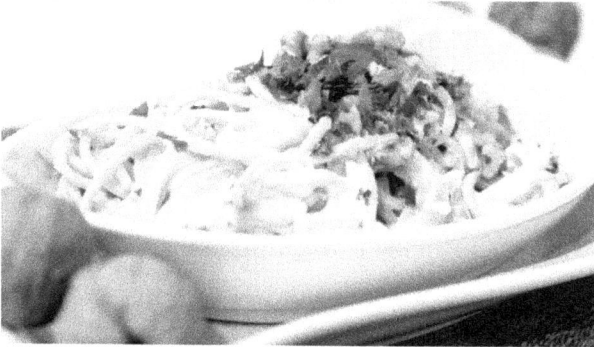

Recipe ID card

- ~ 290 Kcal calories per serving
- ~ Difficulty very easy
- ~ Serves 2
- ~ Preparation 15 minutes
- ~ Low cost

Ingredients

- ~ 160 g of whole wheat spaghetti or whole wheat pasta
- ~ 80 g of vegetable cream
- ~ 50 g of walnut kernels
- ~ grated rind of untreated lemon
- ~ salt
- ~ pepper
- ~ 1 sprig of parsley

Material Required

- ~ Casserole with lid for cooking pasta
- ~ Frying pan for the sauce
- ~ Carving fork
- ~ Chopping board for food
- ~ Knife preferably ceramic for parsley
- ~ Knife
- ~ Nutcracker

Preparation

Bring water to a boil in a large saucepan. Season with salt. When boiling, plunge in the whole wheat spaghetti and cook for 10 minutes (check the package for optimal cooking time).

Meanwhile, prepare the accompanying sauce. Crush the walnuts with the walnut press and coarsely chop the kernels.

Heat the vegetable cream over very low heat: grate the zest of half an organic lemon and continue stirring. If desired, add a few drops of lemon juice to obtain a sauce with a stronger flavor.

Drain the pasta al dente and finish cooking it in the cream and lemon sauce. If necessary, add a ladleful of pasta cooking water: the sauce should not be too dry.

Chop the parsley and add it to the pasta. Serve the pasta steaming hot with pepper and chopped walnuts.

Chickpea soup

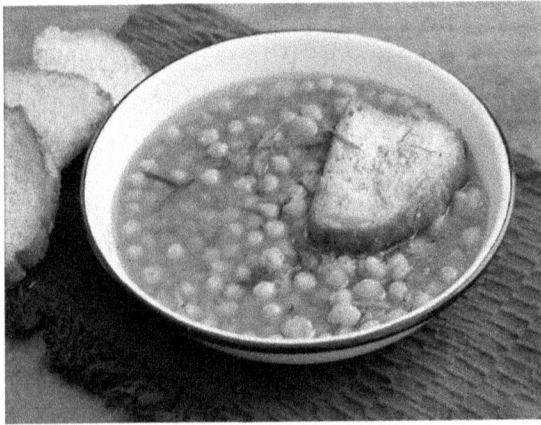

Recipe ID card

- ~ 91 Kcal calories per serving
- ~ Easy difficulty
- ~ Serves 4
- ~ Preparation 90 minutes
- ~ Low cost
- ~ 90 minutes for cooking (chickpeas must soak at least 24 hours)

Ingredients

For the soup

- ~ 1 celery leg
- ~ 2 sage leaves
- ~ salt
- ~ 1 sprig of rosemary
- ~ pepper
- ~ 50 g (one slice) fresh bacon
- ~ 200 g of chickpeas
- ~ 150 g (one medium) carrots
- ~ (about 1.5 l) water

To serve

- ~ a few slices of bread

Material Required

- ~ 1 bowl for soaking chickpeas
- ~ 1 wooden spoon for stirring the soup
- ~ 1 ladle
- ~ 1 mixer (optional)
- ~ 1 chopping board
- ~ 1 sharp knife
- ~ 1 saucepan with lid for cooking the soup
- ~ 1 pot for boiling chickpeas

Preparation

First of all, soak the chickpeas in abundant water. Chickpeas must never be uncovered, therefore it is recommended to add some water in case there is little liquid.

After 24 hours, drain the chickpeas from the soaking water and boil them in abundant salted water for at least 1½ hours.

In the meantime, prepare the seasoning to flavor the soup. In a cutting board, cut the bacon into very thin strips. Dice the celery and carrot as well.

In a saucepan, brown the bacon without adding oil, butter or other seasonings: we will use only the fat of the bacon. When it is well browned, add the chopped celery and carrot and continue cooking for 3-4 minutes, lowering the heat and covering the casserole with the lid. Then turn off the flame.

When the chickpeas are ready, with the aid of a slotted spoon, transfer them to the saucepan containing the vegetables and the bacon, adding 200 ml of cooking water (about 3 ladles). Bring to a boil again, adding some seasonings such as the sage and rosemary.

Those who wish can blend some of the chickpeas with an immersion blender in order to make the soup a bit creamier.

Serve hot with a generous sprinkling of pepper, together with some slices of rustic bread.

Azuki Bean Soup

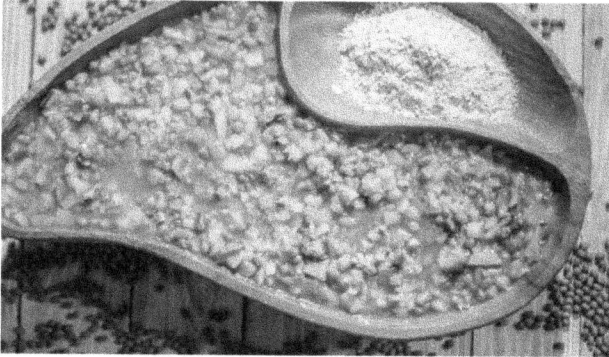

Recipe ID card

- ~ Easy difficulty
- ~ Serves 4
- ~ Preparation 15 minutes
- ~ Low cost
- ~ 15 minutes for preparation; 30 minutes for cooking

Ingredients

- ~ 150 g of adzuki beans
- ~ 120 g of carrots
- ~ 120 g of zucchini
- ~ 200 g of potatoes
- ~ 10 g of dried mushrooms
- ~ about 1 l of water
- ~ 1 piece of kombu seaweed
- ~ Optional: 10 g of brewer's yeast flakes
- ~ If necessary: 1 pinch of salt

Material Required

- ~ Vegetable peeler
- ~ Chopping board
- ~ Casserole with lid
- ~ Scissors

Preparation

Wash the vegetables and dry them with a cloth. Peel the potato and carrot, cut them into strips and then obtain cubes. Remove the ends from the zucchini and dice them.

Cut the dried mushrooms into very small pieces, using scissors or a knife.

Combine the fresh vegetables and chopped dried mushrooms in a saucepan, then add the green adzuki beans and cover flush with water (about 1 litre).

Cut the Kombu seaweed with scissors and add it to the vegetables.

Bring the pot to a boil, then lower the heat, cover with a lid and cook gently for 20-30 minutes, until the beans are soft. If the liquid dries up too much during cooking, add more hot water or hot vegetable broth.

At the end of the cooking time, taste the soup and, if necessary, adjust the salt.

Serve the bean soup by adding a spoonful or two of yeast flakes: this particular ingredient will give a very particular taste to the soup, which will remind the one of grana cheese.

Beans Soup with Barley

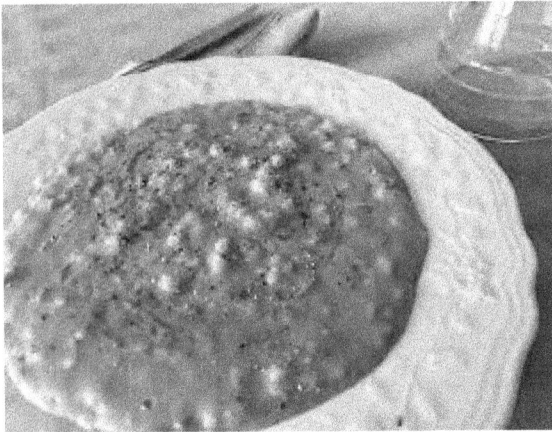

Recipe ID card

- ~ 88 Kcal calories per serving
- ~ Easy difficulty
- ~ Serves 6
- ~ Preparation 90 minutes
- ~ Low cost
- ~ 1 1/2 hours for cooking; 12 hours for soaking beans

Ingredients

- ~ 200 g of dried beans
- ~ A few sage leaves
- ~ Salt
- ~ 100 g of peeled tomatoes or canned tomatoes
- ~ 1 pinch of chilli pepper
- ~ 100 g (1 medium) of carrots
- ~ 2 tablespoons of extra virgin olive oil
- ~ 1 clove of garlic
- ~ 200 g of pearl barley
- ~ 1 celery stalk

Material Required

- ~ Soaking bowl
- ~ 2 Casseroles with lids
- ~ Blender
- ~ Vegetable peeler
- ~ Wooden spoon or ladle

Preparation

Soak the dried beans in plenty of cold water. Leave them to soak overnight (10-12 hours).

Rinse the beans from the soaking water in order to eliminate all the anti-nutritional substances, then boil them for about an hour and a half, until they become soft. Once ready, drain the beans keeping the cooking liquid aside.

In the meantime, cook pearl barley in lightly salted water for 20 minutes or until beans are soft. Drain the water and set aside.

Then prepare the sauce. Clean and wash carrot and celery thoroughly; cut vegetables into pieces and chop finely in a blender.

Brown the chopped celery and carrot in a casserole, adding a drizzle of oil, a clove of garlic, the peeled tomatoes and sage. Season with salt. Those who wish can spice up the sauce with hot pepper.

Flavor the beans in the sauce, add the pearl barley and cover with the cooking liquid from the beans. Boil for about ten minutes.

Serve the soup hot, accompanying it with some rustic bread.

Main courses for diabetics

Fake Ricotta cheese

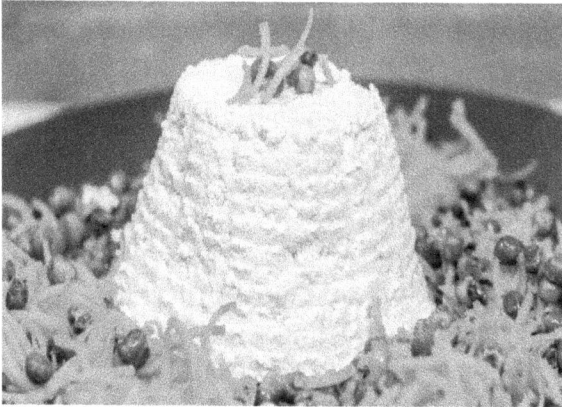

Recipe ID card

~ Easy difficulty
~ Serves 4
~ Preparation 20 minutes
~ Low cost

Ingredients

For about 250 g of ricotta

~ 2 litres of UHT whole milk or pasteurized whole milk
~ 4 tablespoons (40 ml) of rice vinegar
~ 2 tablespoons (20 ml) vinegar
~ salt

Material Required

~ Fuscella
~ Dishcloth
~ Sieve
~ Skimmer
~ Food thermometer
~ Wooden spoon

Preparation

Pour the whole milk into a saucepan and bring to 80°C.

In the meantime, line a colander with a clean dish towel, then place it over a bowl.

When the milk reaches temperature, slowly pour in the rice vinegar and white wine vinegar a little at a time.

Continue stirring with a wooden spoon: you will notice the formation of white clots. As they come to the surface, remove the milk flakes with a skimmer and put them in a dishcloth placed over the strainer.

Proceed in this way until no more flakes are visible in the milk.

Leave the ricotta to drain in the dishcloth, avoiding exerting excessive pressure: the ricotta should not be too dry.

At this time, salt the ricotta to taste, and stir to distribute the salt evenly: the ricotta will take about 5 minutes to drain.

At this point, remove the ricotta from the cloth with a spoon or ladle and, for a better presentation, place it in a "fuscella".

Press gently to give the classic shape of the ricotta, then turn the pan over.

Ricotta is ready: it can be tasted hot or left to cool in the refrigerator and served cold.

Ricotta can be kept in the refrigerator for 2-3 days. Freezing is not recommended.

Roast Pork with Oranges

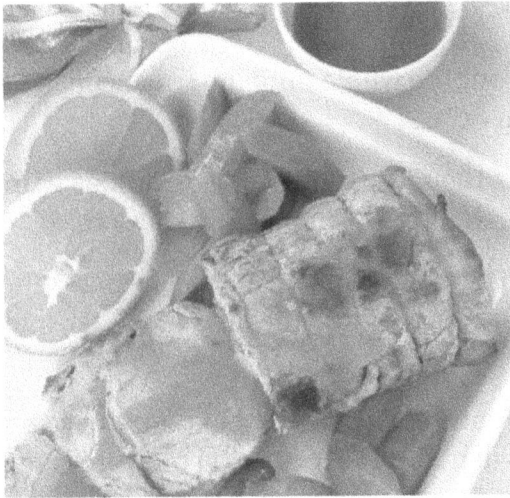

Recipe ID card

~ 80 Kcal calories per serving
~ Easy difficulty
~ Serves 4
~ Preparation 120 minutes
~ Low cost
~ About 2 hours for cooking + cooling time

Ingredients

For the roast

~ 500 g pork loin
~ 4-5 stars (fruits) of aniseed
~ 20 g of brown sugar
~ pepper
~ salt
~ about 150 ml of red wine
~ Grated zest and 150 ml of untreated orange juice

For serving

~ 4-5 stars (fruits) of aniseed
~ about 400 g (2 large) untreated oranges
~ 150 g of spicy mustard

Material Required

~ Cutting board
~ Casserole with lid
~ Sharp knife/slicer
~ Orange peel grater
~ Juicer

Preparation

Cut an orange in half and squeeze its juice. About 150 ml of juice should be obtained.

Leave a pot on the stove and, when it is very hot, brown the pork loin (or loin) on all sides. This will take 3-4 minutes.

When the meat is well browned, add the brown sugar and blend with the red wine. Also add the orange juice and grated orange zest, and the aniseed (stars).

Bring to the boil over high heat. Continue cooking over a gentle heat for about a couple of hours, until the meat is tender. It is advisable to check the roast often during cooking to prevent the liquid from evaporating excessively: if this should happen, it is recommended to add more liquid, making sure not to let it come to a boil.

Salt and pepper the meat to taste 5 minutes before removing the roast from the heat.

Remove the meat from the pot and allow it to cool completely.

Once cooled, cut the roast into 4-5 mm thin slices (recommended to use a slicer). Serve the roast slices in a serving dish, alternating orange slices, orange zest and anise stars. If you like contrasts, you can serve the roast accompanied by spicy mustard pieces.

Ceviche

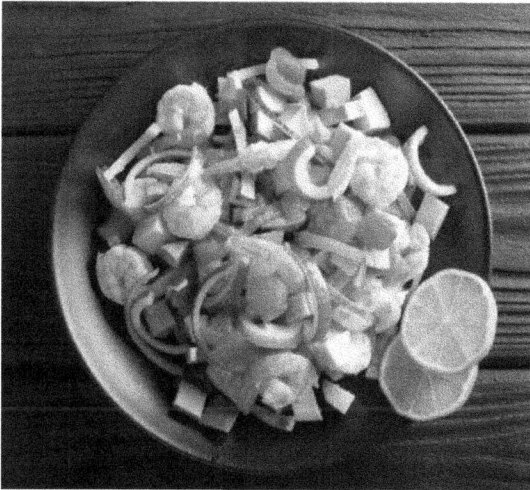

Recipe ID card

- ~ 84 Kcal calories per serving
- ~ Easy difficulty
- ~ Serves 2
- ~ Preparation 20 minutes
- ~ Average cost
- ~ 20 minutes for preparation; 30 minutes for marinade

Ingredients

- ~ 250 g of perch
- ~ 50 g of corn
- ~ 100 g of fried peppers
- ~ 100 g of tomatoes or cherry tomatoes
- ~ 1 clove of garlic
- ~ salt
- ~ 60 ml of pink grapefruit juice
- ~ 15 ml untreated lemon juice
- ~ 15 ml of lime juice
- ~ A few stems of chives

Material Required

- ~ Cutting board
- ~ Knife
- ~ Bowls of various sizes
- ~ Transparent film
- ~ Juicer

Preparation

After thermally chilling the fish, proceed with marinating. Cut the raw fish into small bites and place them in a glass or ceramic bowl. Avoid using aluminium or copper bowls because they may give an unpleasant aftertaste to the fish.

Prepare the marinade. Squeeze the juice from the citrus fruits (lime, lemon and pink grapefruit, in this case) and distribute it over the fish. Season with salt and a clove of garlic, whole or chopped, and chopped chives.

Cover the raw fish with cling film and leave to marinate for at least half an hour.

Drain fish from excess marinade. Briefly heat the corn in a pan, without adding seasonings. Cut the friggitelli into rounds, the celery into small pieces and the tomatoes into slices.

Serve the ceviche with the hot corn, slices of friggitelli, celery and tomato.

Cotechino and Lentils

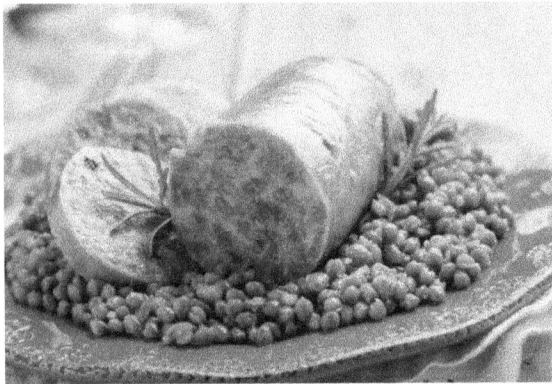

Recipe ID card

~ 211 Kcal calories per serving
~ Difficulty fairly easy
~ Serves 8
~ Preparation 210 minutes
~ Average cost
~ 2 hours for cooking cotechino; 90 minutes for cooking lentils; 12 hours for soaking

Ingredients

~ 1 garlic clove
~ salt
~ pepper
~ 2 tablespoons of extra virgin olive oil
~ 250 g of dried lentils
~ Gluten-free product: 600 g of cotechino
~ 1 tablespoon of tomato paste
~ 150 g of carrots
~ 500 ml vegetable stock
~ 1 bay leaf
~ Some celery ribs

Material Required

~ Bowl
~ Saucepan with lid
~ Blender
~ Pot with steamer basket
~ Serving dish
~ Cutting board
~ Sharp knife

Preparation

First, soak the lentils. Pour the dried legumes into a large bowl and cover with plenty of cold water. Leave the lentils to soak for at least 10-12 hours, until they have tripled their volume.

Just before starting the preparation of the lentils, steam the cotechino for at least 3 hours.

At this point, rinse the lentils in cold water to remove all of the anti-nutritional elements contained in the seeds.

Clean the vegetables: wash and peel the carrots and cut them into small pieces. Wash the celery and cut it into small pieces. Chop the vegetables in a mixer.

Brown the chopped vegetables in a saucepan, adding 2 tablespoons of oil, a tablespoon of tomato paste and a clove of garlic.

Pour the rinsed lentils into a saucepan and cover the surface with the hot vegetable stock. Cook for 1 1/2 to 2 hours, depending on the type of lentils chosen. It is recommended to check the lentils often during cooking: if the liquid evaporates too much, add a few more ladles of broth.

When the lentils are soft, add salt and pepper to taste and season with a bay leaf. Continue cooking for another 5 minutes.

Remove the cotechino from the steamer basket and cut into the surface: the casing will come off very easily.

Cut the cotechino into slices and serve with the lentils. This dish is also great paired with mashed potatoes.

Green Pepper Fillet LIGHT

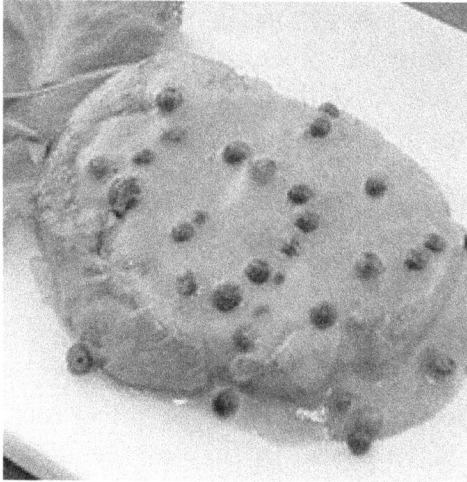

Recipe ID card

- ~ 130 Kcal calories per serving
- ~ Easy difficulty
- ~ Serves 2
- ~ Preparation 15 minutes
- ~ High cost

Ingredients

- ~ 2 pieces of 150 g each of beef fillet
- ~ 150 g of fresh ricotta
- ~ 50-60 ml of skimmed milk
- ~ 1 generous spoonful of green pepper in brine
- ~ 1 pinch of salt
- ~ 1 teaspoon of mustard

Material Required

- ~ Saucepan
- ~ Pan with lid
- ~ Mortar or meat pestle (for crushing pepper)
- ~ Dustpan or tongs
- ~ Serving dish

Preparation

First crush a part of green pepper (well drained from the brine) with a mortar or a meat pounder.

Heat a little milk in a saucepan and add the partially crushed green peppercorns and mustard. Cook over a very gentle flame for 2-3 minutes.

Remove from the heat and add the ricotta: mix well to form a cream. If necessary, add more milk. It is recommended not to cook the sauce to keep it liquid.

Heat a pan on the stove, not too large, and cover with a lid. After a couple of minutes, remove the lid and brown the fillets 2 minutes per side, keeping a lively flame. Do not add oil or butter: the heat of the pan will be enough for an inviting crust to form on the meat. Brown the meat on the sides as well to maintain the classic regular shape of the fillet.

When browning is complete, lower the heat, add salt to taste, cover with the lid and continue cooking for a further 2 minutes (medium-cooking of the fillet). Those who like their tenderloin "rare" can avoid this step.

With the heat off, add the ricotta and green pepper sauce directly to the pan. Cover with the lid a couple of minutes and serve immediately.

Vegetable Fillet with Green Pepper

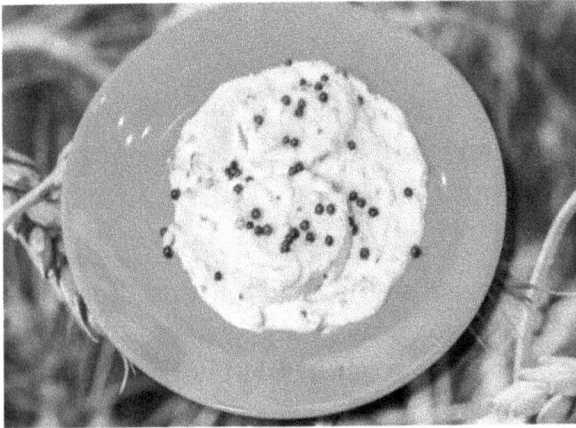

Recipe ID card

- ~ 288 Kcal calories per serving
- ~ Difficulty fairly easy
- ~ Serves 4
- ~ Preparation 15 minutes
- ~ Average cost

Ingredients

- ~ 80 ml of soy milk
- ~ 200 g or 3 slices of muscle wheat
- ~ 100 ml of corn seed oil
- ~ 1 tablespoon of extra virgin olive oil
- ~ 1 heaped tablespoon of green pepper in brine
- ~ 1 pinch of salt
- ~ 1 teaspoon of mustard

Material Required

- ~ Immersion mixer + beaker
- ~ Pan with lid
- ~ Mortar (optional)
- ~ Tongs or spatula
- ~ Pasta cup or cookie cutter (optional)

Preparation

Cut the wheat muscle into 1.5 cm thick slices. To improve the aesthetics of the dish, make regular medallions of vegetable meat using a pasta cutter or a cookie cutter.

Pour a drizzle of extra virgin olive oil in a pan and brown the wheat muscle well, adding salt to taste.

Crush the green peppercorns in a mortar or with a simple spoon and pour them into a saucepan along with 30 ml of soy milk and mustard paste. In this way, you can enhance the spicy aroma of the pepper. Cook for 5 minutes.

Prepare the vegetable cream: pour 50 ml soy milk into a beaker and add 100 ml vegetable oil.

Dissolve the resulting vegetable cream in the saucepan of pepper-flavoured soy milk.

Turn off the wheat muscle pan and pour in the vegetable sauce. Cover with the lid and allow the sauce to dry.

Serve the green pepper veggie tenderloin piping hot.

Homemade Milk Flakes

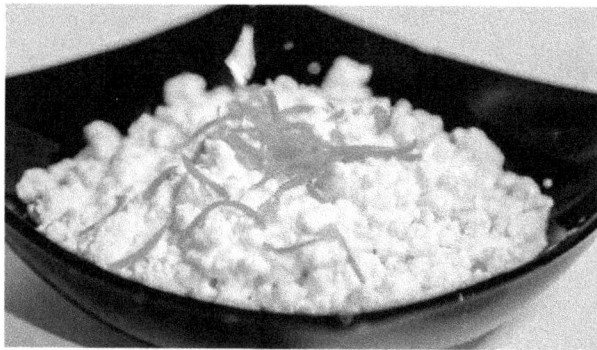

Recipe ID card

~ Difficulty quite easy
~ Serves 2
~ Preparation 100 minutes
~ Low cost
~ 20 minutes preparation + 80 minutes rest

Ingredients

~ 2 l of pasteurized skimmed milk or semi-skimmed milk
~ 1 g of rennet powder
~ 10 ml of water
~ 1 pinch of salt (optional)
~ Optional: 50 g natural yoghurt or fresh cream

Material Required

~ Large saucepan with lid
~ Bowls of different sizes
~ Wooden spoon
~ Fine-mesh sieve or dish towel
~ Pasta strainer (if necessary)
~ Thermometer
~ Long blade knife
~ Latex gloves
~ Skimmer or whisk

Preparation

Pour the pasteurized skim milk into a saucepan and warm until it reaches 30°C (86°F). Turn off the heat.

Dissolve rennet powder in 10 ml of warm water. When it has solubilized, pour the rennet into the warm milk and stir with a wooden spoon for a couple of minutes.

Close the saucepan with the lid and wait one hour without stirring.

After an hour, the curd will have formed. Insert a long-bladed knife into the curd. Make some crossed cuts in order to form some squares or rhombuses with an approximate side of 4 cm: it should be obtained a sort of grid.

Wait 10 minutes to facilitate the hardening of the curd and its detachment from the whey.

Light the fire and heat the curdled milk very slowly, continuing to stir in order to avoid the cubes of curd to stick together. Bring everything to 51-53°C.

Wait 10 minutes again to allow the curds to settle to the bottom.

Stir the milk flakes still dispersed in the whey, trying to remove them with a skimmer or a whisk.

Drain milk flakes on a colander or on a clean cloth placed over a colander. If necessary, remove the flakes of milk with your hands (possibly protected by gloves). Let the milk flakes drip for half an hour.

Those who want a creamier texture can add some spoons of milk cream (fresh cream) or yogurt for a lighter version.

Milky flakes can be stored in the refrigerator for 3-4 days, in a bowl covered with plastic wrap.

Chickpea Burger

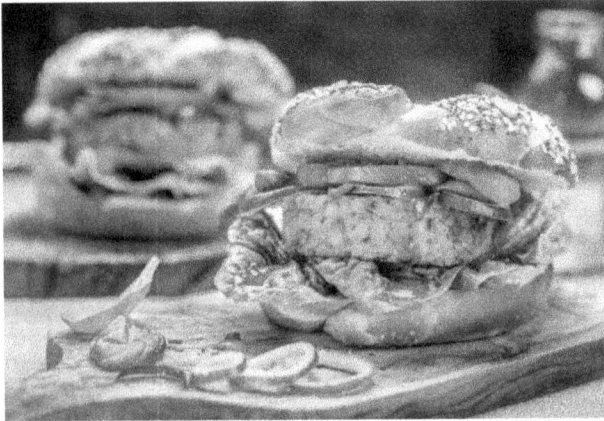

~ Electric blender

~ Scoop

Preparation

Blend the boiled chickpeas (drained from the cooking water) together with a few tablespoons of vegetable milk (e.g. soy milk or rice milk), a tablespoon of olive oil and the tofu, until a thick cream is obtained.

Mix the chickpea cream with salt and spices (chili pepper, paprika, ginger). If you wish, you can also add a teaspoon of sweet mustard. Add the organic potato flakes until the mixture is easily mouldable. In case the dough is too thick, add another tablespoon of vegetable milk.

Roll out the dough on the pastry board, with the help of a rolling pin: you should obtain a sheet about 1 cm thick.

With the round pastry cutter, obtain 6 or 7 veggie burgers.

Heat 2 tablespoons of oil in a frying pan and brown the burgers for 2 minutes on each side. Lower the heat, cover with the lid and cook for another 5 minutes. Serve the chickpea burgers with fresh vegetables, adding a few drops of lemon if desired.

Recipe ID card

~ 214 Kcal calories per serving
~ Easy difficulty
~ Serves 3
~ Preparation 20 minutes
~ Low cost

Ingredients

For about 6-8 chickpea burgers

~ Ready-made product: 250 g chickpeas
~ 50 g of tofu
~ Organic product: 25 g potato flakes
~ 4-5 tablespoons of soy milk
~ salt
~ 1 pinch of chili pepper
~ 1 teaspoon of sweet paprika
~ 1 teaspoon of ginger
~ 3 tablespoons extra virgin olive oil

Material Required

~ Bowl
~ Flattener
~ Round mold with a diameter of 8 cm
~ Pan with lid
~ Wooden spoon

Soy and Rice Hamburger

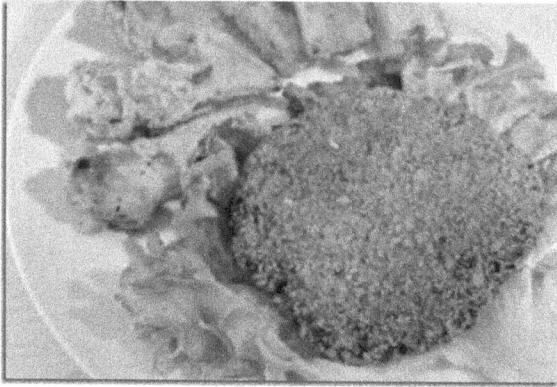

Recipe ID card

~ 148 Kcal calories per serving
~ Difficulty fairly easy
~ Serves 8
~ Preparation 80 minutes
~ Low cost
~ 1 hour cooking time for soybeans; 15 minutes for burger preparation; 5 minutes cooking time + soaking time for soybeans (12 hours)

Ingredients

For 8-10 soy burgers

~ 100 g of yellow soybeans
~ 2 tablespoons of extra virgin olive oil
~ 1 tablespoon of soy sauce
~ 1 pinch of salt
~ 1 teaspoon of sweet paprika
~ 1 sprig of parsley
~ a few leaves of sage
~ about 60 g of breadcrumbs
~ about 50 ml of soy milk
~ about 150 g (2 medium-sized) carrots
~ 80 g brown rice

Optional: to accompany

~ salt
~ 1 handful of arugula
~ 100 g cucumbers
~ 100 g (1.5 oz) coppery tomatoes
~ 150 g (1 medium) of peppers
~ half a small glass of untreated lemon juice

Material Required

~ Large bowl for soaking soybeans
~ Dough bowl
~ Chopping board or pastry board
~ Mold (bowl or cup)
~ Casserole for cooking legumes
~ Saucepan for cooking rice
~ Immersion blender with high-sided container
~ Vegetable peeler for carrots
~ Stone or non-stick pan for cooking burgers
~ Scoop
~ Knife

Preparation

Soak the yellow soybeans in a very large bowl for 12-24 hours, until they have doubled in volume.

Rinse the soybeans in cold water, then transfer them to a saucepan full of water (adding a pinch of salt) and cook for about 60-80 minutes, until soft.

Wash and peel the carrots, then boil them in plenty of lightly salted water.

Also boil the brown rice in salted water for 20-30 minutes.

When the soybeans, carrots and brown rice are ready, proceed with shaping the burgers.

Pour the cooked soybeans into a beaker, add the carrots and soy milk. Mix everything until you get a very thick mixture.

Pour the resulting cream into a bowl, add the boiled rice, chopped parsley, sage, soy sauce and enough breadcrumbs to make a fairly compact mixture that can be shaped by hand.

Pour a layer of breadcrumbs on a surface and spread the mixture until it is about 1.5 cm thick.

Cover again with breadcrumbs and obtain 8-10 discs by cutting the dough with a round pasta cup or the edge of a cup.

Pour 2 tablespoons of oil into a large frying pan: when hot, brown the burgers on both sides and continue cooking for 5 minutes.

Meanwhile, prepare the accompanying vegetables. Cut the bell pepper, tomato and cucumber into cubes: season with a little salt, a little extra virgin olive oil and a dash of lemon.

Accompany the soy burgers with the vegetable salad and arugula leaves.

Chicken and Avocado Salad

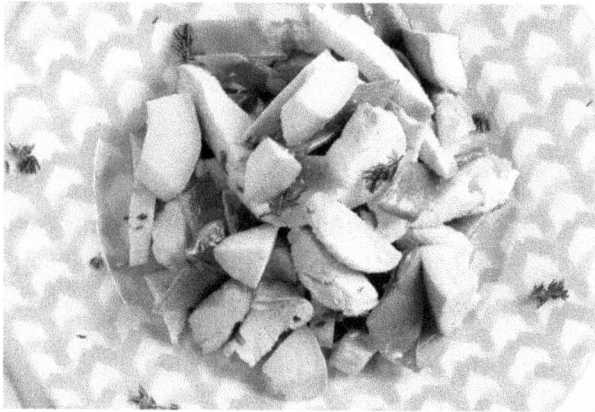

Recipe ID card

- ~ 114 Kcal calories per serving
- ~ Easy difficulty
- ~ Serves 2
- ~ Preparation 15 minutes
- ~ Average cost
- ~ 15 minutes + cooling time of mayonnaise

Ingredients

For the chicken salad

- ~ 300 g of chicken breast
- ~ 2 tablespoons of extra virgin olive oil
- ~ 1 teaspoon of ginger
- ~ 1 teaspoon of sweet paprika
- ~ of salt
- ~ 30 g black olives
- ~ 1 rib of celery
- ~ a few leaves of mint
- ~ 1 tuft of parsley
- ~ half a small glass of untreated lemon juice
- ~ 250 g of avocado

For the oil-free vegetable mayonnaise

- ~ 3 stalks of chives
- ~ 30 g capers
- ~ 20 g of egg yolks

- ~ 1 teaspoon of mustard
- ~ 5 ml vinegar
- ~ 1 tablespoon untreated lemon juice
- ~ 1 pinch of salt
- ~ 180 ml water
- ~ 14 g rice flour
- ~ 30 g gherkins

Material Required

- ~ Knife digger
- ~ Knife
- ~ Cutting board
- ~ Frying pan
- ~ Mayonnaise saucepan
- ~ Mayonnaise blender
- ~ Blender

Preparation

Prepare the light mayonnaise without oil, whose specific recipe is given in this video.

Pour the gherkins, chives and capers into a blender until they form a fairly thick cream. Add the vegetable mixture to the refrigerated mayonnaise.

Grill the chicken breast on a stone or non-stick griddle, adding salt to taste. Cook for a few minutes, covering the pan with a lid.

In the meantime, prepare the avocado: cut the fruit in half, remove the central stone and, with the digger, obtain many small balls.

Cut the chicken into thin slices or cubes, and pour into a bowl. Add the avocado balls, olives, chopped celery and season with chopped parsley and mint, sweet paprika, ginger and black olives.

Fill an avocado shell with the chicken salad and serve topped with the vegetable mayonnaise.

Turkey Rolls

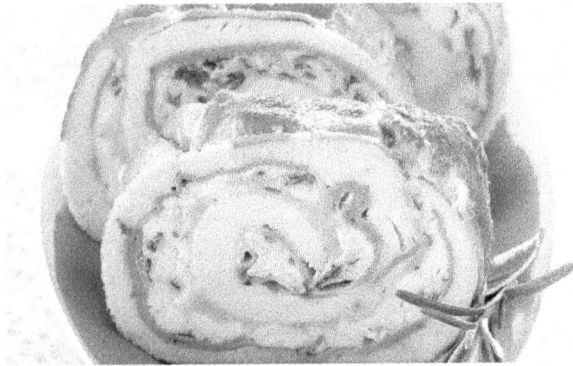

Recipe ID card

~ 107 Kcal calories per serving
~ Easy difficulty
~ Serves 2
~ Preparation 15 minutes
~ Low cost

Ingredients

For 6 rolls

~ 6 slices (120 g) of turkey rump
~ A few stalks of chives
~ A few basil leaves
~ A few leaves of lettuce or salad greens
~ 20 g of gomasio
~ 200 g of fresh ricotta cheese

For the accompanying sauce

~ 125 g low-fat yoghurt
~ 1 teaspoon of mustard
~ A few mint leaves
~ Salt

Material Required

~ Cutting board
~ Knives preferably ceramic
~ Immersion mixer
~ Becker
~ Bowl
~ Wooden spoon

Preparation

Prepare the filling for the rolls. In a bowl, mix the fresh ricotta (sifted if necessary) with the gomasio and chopped basil.

Spread a salad leaf (e.g. lettuce) on a thin slice of cooked turkey rump and stuff with a strip of flavored ricotta. Roll up the slice and seal with a stem of chives.

Proceed in this way until all the turkey slices have been used up.

Now prepare the accompanying sauce. In a beaker, combine the low-fat natural yogurt, a few mint leaves, a teaspoon of mustard and a pinch of salt. Blend with an immersion blender until a sauce is obtained.

Serve the rolls, whole or in halves, with the mint sauce.

Homemade Mozzarella

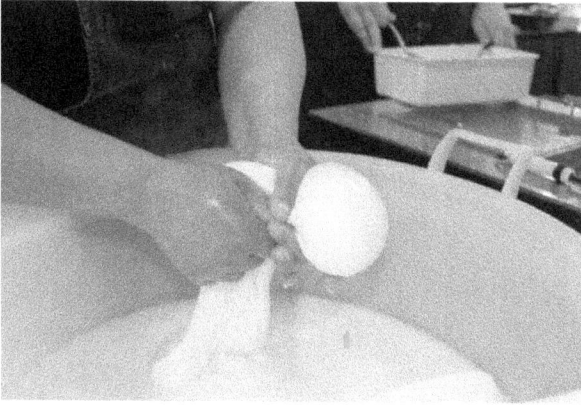

Recipe ID card

~ Very difficult
~ Serves 10 people
~ Preparation 210 minutes
~ Average cost

Ingredients

For the mozzarella

~ 3 liters of raw milk
~ 4 g of citric acid
~ 50 ml of water
~ 1.2 ml (36 drops) of liquid rennet

For the brine

~ 1 L of water
~ 8 g of coarse salt

Material Required

~ Food thermometer (essential)
~ Very large saucepan
~ Long blade knife
~ Whisk
~ Ladle
~ Bowls of various sizes
~ Pasta strainer
~ Saucepan
~ Latex gloves (optional)

Preparation

Heat raw milk to 70-72°C and hold this temperature for 3-5 minutes.

Cool the pasteurized milk to a temperature of 15°C. Dissolve the citric acid in 50 ml of water, then slowly add it to the cold milk, continuing to stir for a couple of minutes.

Warm the milk until it reaches 33-36°C: turn off the flame and slowly add the liquid rennet a little at a time.

Let the curd rest for an hour.

It is now possible to proceed with the first breaking of the curd. With a long-bladed knife make cross cuts in the curd until a grid is formed. It is advisable to make diamond shapes of about 4 cm per side.

Let the curd rest for 10-15 minutes, in order to facilitate the detachment from the whey.

You can now proceed with the second breaking. Dip a whisk (or a skimmer) in the curd, until the mass is broken. The "grains" of curd should be the size of a peanut.

Let the curd rest for another 15 minutes, in order to facilitate again the detachment from the whey and the hardening.

After 15 minutes, the curd will have settled on the bottom. Remove slowly and little by little the whey with the help of a ladle: in this way, curd will be slowly dried by its whey.

Once most of the whey has been removed, remove the curd from the saucepan and gently tip it in a pan, in order to remove as much whey as possible. In order to facilitate the operation, it is also advisable to break the curd with hands or with a knife.

Proceed with the spinning test. Heat water in a small saucepan until it reaches 80-85°C (176-185°F): remove a fragment of curd from the mass and place it in a small bowl. Pour the very hot water and mix with a stick or the tip of a knife: if the curd has reached the right acidity (5.6-5.8), the fragment taken should form a long thread or be very elastic and moldable.

If the spinning test has been successful, then it is possible to proceed with the actual spinning. Pour the curd in a steel bowl and slowly add water at a temperature of 80-85° C (176-85° F) little by little. Mozzarella must be worked with delicacy and wrapped on itself as the paste is spinning. The cheese must be often dipped in hot water until the progressive hardening of the mass is perceived.

At this point, the dough is ready to be cut: squeeze the dough between hands and twist the obtained strand until smooth and regular balls are obtained.

Store mozzarellas in the 50:50 preserving liquid, that is in a solution prepared with 1 part of water and 1 part of whey.

Vegan Mozzarella Cheese

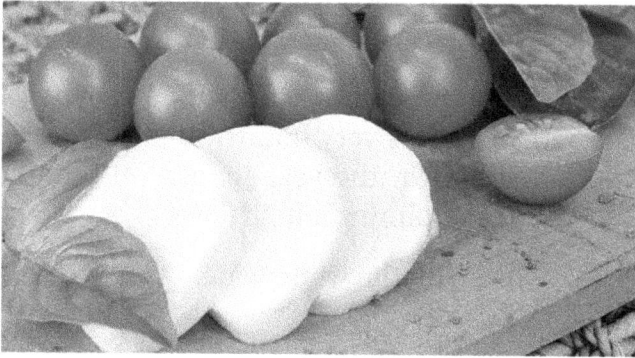

Recipe ID card

- 224 Kcal calories per serving
- Easy difficulty
- Serves 2
- Preparation 15 minutes
- Low cost
- 15 minutes + 1 hour cooling time

Ingredients

For the vegetable mozzarella

- 50 g of cornflour or potato starch
- 60 ml + 2 tablespoons of soy milk
- 70 g of soy yogurt
- 4 tablespoons of corn seed oil
- 1 pinch of salt

To accompany

- 50 g of cherry tomatoes
- 1 pinch of pepper
- 1 drop of extra virgin olive oil
- a few basil leaves
- 1 pinch of salt

Material Required

- Casserole
- Whip
- Precision scale
- Small bowl
- Transparent film
- Chopping board
- Knife
- Immersion mixer and beaker

Preparation

Make a sort of vegetable cream by pouring 2 tablespoons of soy milk and 4 tablespoons of corn seed oil into a beaker. Mix everything with an immersion blender until a slightly thick sauce is obtained.

In a small saucepan, mix the corn-starch, unsweetened soy milk, plain soy yogurt, a pinch of salt and the resulting vegetable cream. Mix with a whisk or a wooden spoon until you get a thick cream.

Place the saucepan on the heat and continue stirring. When the temperature of the mixture increases, the first lumps will form: this phase is absolutely normal. By continuing to stir, the lumps will disappear and you will get a compact ball.

Oil a small bowl with some seed oil and distribute the obtained vegan mozzarella. Cover with plastic wrap and let cool completely.

Serve the mozzarella well chilled, cut into slices, perhaps accompanied with basil, oil, cherry tomatoes and a pinch of salt.

Bone hole ligth

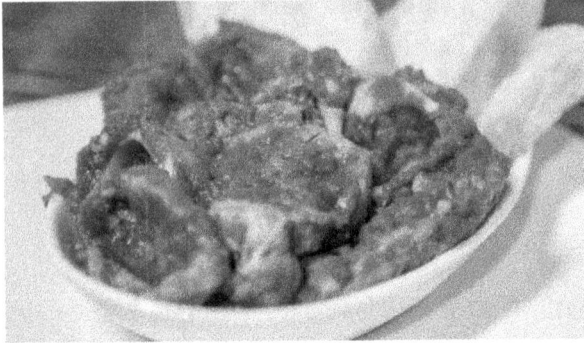

Recipe ID card

- ~ 74 Kcal calories per serving
- ~ Easy difficulty
- ~ Serves 4
- ~ Preparation 100 minutes
- ~ Average cost

Ingredients

- ~ 4 veal or beef shanks (300 g each)
- ~ about 100 ml of dry white wine
- ~ 1 garlic clove
- ~ salt
- ~ pepper
- ~ 400 g of pulp or tomato puree

Material Required

- ~ Knife or scissors
- ~ Frying pan with lid
- ~ Spoon
- ~ Scoop

Preparation

First, cut through the white skin that surrounds the meat: in this way, the ossobuco will not curl during cooking.

Remove the marrow that is in the center of each ossobuco by exerting light pressure. If the marrow struggles to be removed, it is advisable to score it with a knife before pressing.

Heat a stone, steel or non-stick frying pan very hot: when it is very hot, without adding oil or butter, brown the veal shanks on both sides while maintaining a high flame.

Deglaze with the white wine.

Season with salt and pepper to taste. Add a clove of poached or minced garlic (for a more intense flavor).

At this point, add the tomato pulp and keep a lively flame until it comes to a boil.

At this point, lower the heat, cover with the lid and cook slowly for about an hour and a half or until the meat is tender. If necessary, add a little water or broth during cooking.

Serve the bone hole with mashed potatoes or soft polenta.

Salt Fish

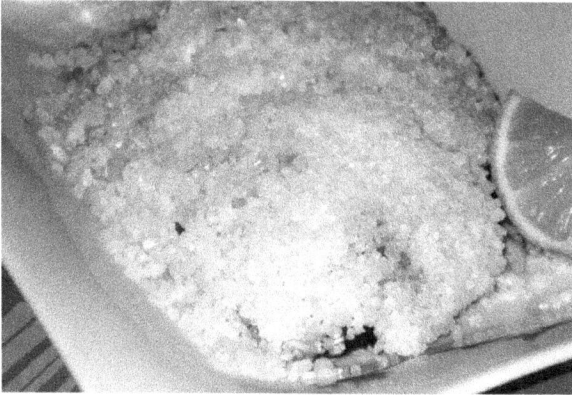

Recipe ID card

~ 89 Kcal calories per serving
~ Easy difficulty
~ Serves 2
~ Preparation 50 minutes
~ Average cost
~ 15 minutes to prepare; 40 minutes to cook

Ingredients

~ 1 clove or 1 teaspoon of garlic powder
~ 120 g (3 medium) egg white
~ Untreated lemon juice
~ 500 g of sea bream
~ 1 sprig of parsley
~ 1 sprig of rosemary
~ About 800 g of salt
~ A few leaves of sage
~ 1 teaspoon of thyme

Material Required

~ Food cutting board
~ Sharp knife
~ Electric whisk
~ Baking tray
~ Mixer or herb knife
~ Latex gloves (optional)

~ Ice-breaker, hammer or meat tenderizer to break up the salt crust
~ Serving dish

Preparation

First clean the fish: remove the fins and incise the belly to remove the entrails. Rinse the fish in running water.

Whip the egg whites until stiff, adding a pinch of salt.

In the meantime, chop the herb mix with a mixer or a knife.

Fill the belly of the fish with a spoonful of the herbs, adding a few drops of lemon too.

Pour the fine salt into a large bowl, add the remaining chopped herbs and mix everything with the egg whites until stiff.

Pour some of the salt and egg white mixture into the bottom of the baking dish, then place the fish with its skin on top. Cover all the fish with the remaining mixture and bake in a hot oven (200°C) for 40 minutes. Cooking time depends on the size and weight of the fish: the larger the fish, the longer it must be cooked.

Remove the fish from the oven and break the salt crust with an ice-breaker or a meat pounder. It is advisable to immediately remove the fish from the crust in order to avoid the food absorbing too much salt.

The fish is now ready to be eaten.

Chicken Curry

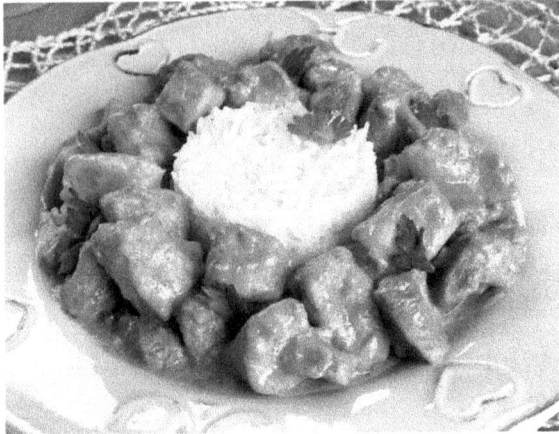

Recipe ID card

- ~ 97 Kcal calories per serving
- ~ Easy difficulty
- ~ Serves 4
- ~ Preparation 20 minutes
- ~ Low cost
- ~ 20 minutes + resting time (1 hour)

Ingredients

- ~ 500 g of chicken breast
- ~ 250 ml low-fat yoghurt
- ~ 2 tablespoons of extra virgin olive oil
- ~ 2 heaped tablespoons of curry powder
- ~ salt
- ~ pepper
- ~ 100 ml of dry white wine
- ~ untreated lemon juice

Material Required

- ~ Bowls of various sizes
- ~ Transparent film
- ~ Frying pan
- ~ Wooden spoon/pallet

Preparation

Cut the chicken breast into cubes. Pour everything into a bowl, adding a drizzle of oil, 1 heaped tablespoon of curry powder, the juice of half a lemon, pepper and salt.

Let the chicken soak for at least an hour to allow it to take on flavor.

After this time has elapsed, heat a frying pan and brown the chicken nuggets.

After browning the chicken, deglaze with the dry white wine and continue cooking over low heat for about 10-15 minutes.

Meanwhile, prepare the accompanying sauce: mix the natural white yogurt with a tablespoon of curry powder.

Once ready, remove the lid from the pan and allow any excess liquid to dry. Remove the pan from the heat and spread the curry yogurt sauce directly over the chicken bites. Close with the lid to let the sauce heat up and flavor the morsels.

Baked Stuffed Chicken

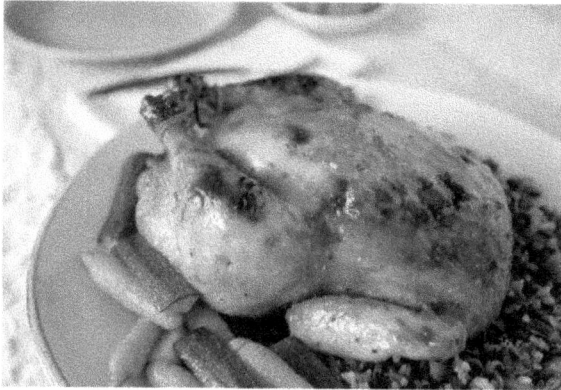

Recipe ID card

- ~ 150 Kcal calories per serving
- ~ Difficulty fairly easy
- ~ Serves 8
- ~ Preparation 130 minutes
- ~ Average cost
- ~ 40 minutes for preparation; 90 minutes for cooking

Ingredients

For the chicken

- ~ 100-150 ml dry white wine
- ~ 1 tablespoon of roasting spices
- ~ A few leaves of sage
- ~ salt
- ~ 1 sprig of rosemary
- ~ 1 garlic clove
- ~ pepper
- ~ 70 g of stale bread
- ~ 100 g of fresh bacon
- ~ 1 grated nutmeg
- ~ 150 ml of milk
- ~ 100 g (1 medium) of carrots
- ~ 500 g of lean mixed minced meat
- ~ 1 Kg of whole chicken

To accompany

- ~ 500 g of potatoes

Material Required

- ~ Bowls of various sizes
- ~ Cooking twine
- ~ Roasting needle
- ~ Latex gloves (optional)
- ~ Baking dish preferably in pyrex
- ~ Ladle or spoon
- ~ Chopping board
- ~ Knife

Preparation

After having boned the chicken well (but leaving the wings for an optimal presentation), you can proceed with the preparation of the stuffing. Cut the stale bread into cubes and soak it in warm milk for about ten minutes.

Transfer the meat and the minced bacon to a bowl: add salt and pepper to taste, add the spice mix, grated nutmeg and the bread squeezed out of the milk. Knead the filling thoroughly until a homogeneous mixture is obtained.

Peel a carrot, wash it and remove the ends.

Fill the chicken - boned and opened - with the flavored mince, taking care to fill the thighs as well. Place the peeled carrot in the center and close the edges of the meat, until the whole chicken is shaped again. We recommend referring to the video.

With the help of a large roasting needle (or a simple sterilized kitchen needle) and a string, sew the edges of the chicken taking care not to stretch the skin too much to avoid breaking it.

Peel the potatoes and cut them into fairly large pieces. Plunge them into cold water.

Place the stuffed and sewn chicken on a baking sheet (which should not be too big!): it is advisable to place the chicken on the baking sheet from the back side (from the side where it has been sewn). Season with salt and pepper to taste. Add a teaspoon of spice mix, sage, rosemary and a clove of garlic. Drizzle the chicken with half a glass of dry white wine.

Cover the chicken with aluminium foil and bake for 30 minutes at 200°C.

After half an hour, remove the pan from the oven, being careful not to burn. If necessary, add white wine: do not use oil!

Drain the potatoes from the water and distribute them in the chicken pan.

Bake the pan again and continue cooking for another hour at 180-200°C. It is advisable to sprinkle the chicken often with the cooking liquid using a spoon.

Vegetarian Quinoa Meatballs

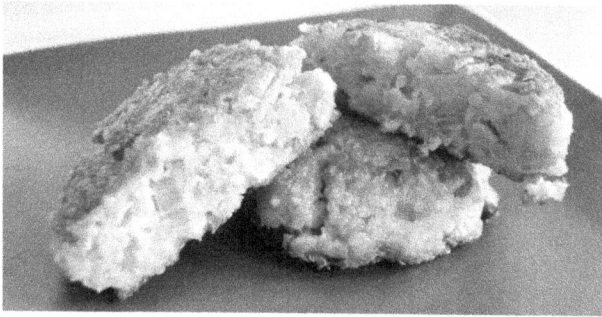

Recipe ID card

~ 185 Kcal calories per serving
~ Difficulty fairly easy
~ Serves 5
~ Preparation 30 minutes
~ Low cost
~ 30 minutes + time for soaking

Ingredients

For about 10 meatballs

~ 150 g of quinoa
~ about 3 tablespoons of extra virgin olive oil
~ 1 sprig of parsley
~ 1 pinch of chili pepper
~ pepper
~ salt
~ Gluten-free product: 70-80 g of breadcrumbs
~ 200 g of radicchio
~ 200 g of cauliflower

To coat

~ Gluten-free product: about 30 g breadcrumbs

Material Required

~ Bowls
~ Casserole
~ Ladle
~ Immersion mixer
~ Pan with lid
~ Plate
~ Chopping board
~ Knife
~ Dense mesh colander/strainer

Preparation

First, thoroughly rinse the dried quinoa in fresh running water.

Cook the quinoa in lightly salted water (the amount of water should be equal to twice the volume of the quinoa). You may want to pour a tablespoon of oil directly into the quinoa cooking water to prevent the seeds from sticking to each other.

Meanwhile, clean the cauliflower and steam it, cutting it into small pieces to speed up cooking time.

Clean the radicchio and cut it into thin strips. Sauté the radicchio in a pan, adding a drizzle of oil, salt and pepper.

Pour the cauliflower into a beaker, add a drizzle of oil, salt, pepper and a couple of tablespoons of quinoa cooking water: blend everything with an immersion blender until you get a cream.

When ready, drain quinoa from water and pour into a bowl. Leave to cool.

Combine cream of cauliflower and radicchio with quinoa and mix thoroughly, seasoning with a little chopped parsley.

Those who wish can also add a pinch of hot pepper to the mixture.

At this point, add a little at a time the gluten-free breadcrumbs (variant for celiac), until the mixture is thick enough to work with your hands. You will need about 70-80 g of gluten-free breadcrumbs.

Cut out the meatballs and roll them in the gluten-free breadcrumbs.

Pour a drop of oil into a frying pan and, when hot, brown the patties: they will be ready in 5 minutes.

Fisherman's clams

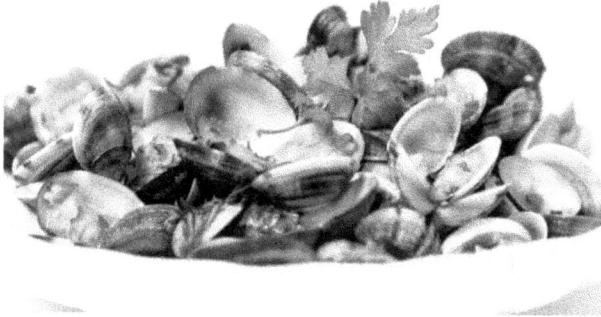

Recipe ID card

- ~ 68 Kcal calories per serving
- ~ Easy difficulty
- ~ Serves 2
- ~ Preparation 145 minutes
- ~ Average cost
- ~ 15 minutes for cleaning; 2 hours for soaking; 10 minutes for cooking

Ingredients

For the soaking

- ~ 1 L of water
- ~ 20 g of salt

For the clams "alla pescatora

- ~ 1 Kg of clams
- ~ 1 tuft of parsley
- ~ half a glass of dry white wine
- ~ 1 tablespoon of extra virgin olive oil
- ~ 1 pinch of pepper
- ~ 1 clove of garlic

Material Required

- ~ Bowls
- ~ Transparent film
- ~ Casserole
- ~ Latex gloves
- ~ Chopping board
- ~ Skimmer
- ~ Wooden ladles or shovels
- ~ Colander
- ~ Strong absorbent paper

Preparation

Before buying clams, it is necessary to make sure the product is certified and guaranteed. Clams must be alive and very fresh: for this reason it is advisable to ascertain the origin and the date they were fished.

Rub the clams with each other and eliminate any open or broken clams, as they could be full of sand.

Beat each clam in a cutting board: in this way, even the most internal sand will be removed.

Prepare a saline solution by dissolving 20 g of coarse salt in 1 litre of water. Plunge the clams and let them soak for a couple of hours, taking care to change the liquid at least a couple of times, until the water will be clear.

Rinse the clams in cold water: now the clams are ready to be cooked as desired.

Heat a dash of oil in a large saucepan and brown a clove of garlic. Add the clams and keep a lively flame. Cover with a lid: the heat will help the shells to hatch.

At this point, add the white wine, season with pepper and continue cooking for 2-3 minutes. Finish with plenty of parsley.

With a skimmer, move the clams to a serving dish or a small bowl.

Strain the sauce by pouring the cooking liquid through a colander lined with heavy-duty paper towels. This will filter out additional grains of sand.

Distribute the strained liquid over the clams and serve immediately.

Stuffed Meat Roll

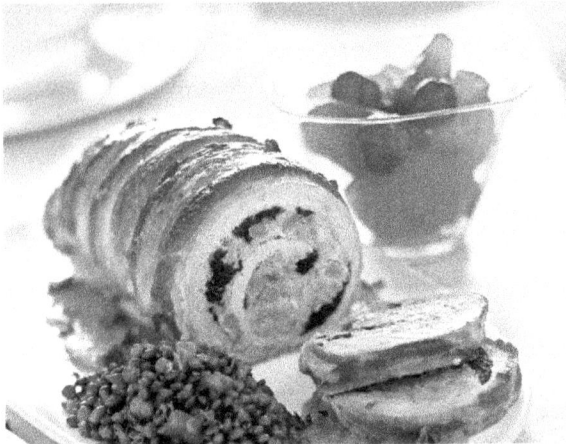

Recipe ID card

- ~ 116 Kcal calories per serving
- ~ Difficulty fairly easy
- ~ Serves 8
- ~ Preparation 120 minutes
- ~ Average cost
- ~ 30 minutes for preparation + 90 minutes for cooking

Ingredients

- ~ 1 bay leaf
- ~ 250 g of spinach
- ~ salt
- ~ 2-3 sage leaves
- ~ 1 sprig of rosemary
- ~ 100 g of cooked ham
- ~ pepper
- ~ For the spinach: 2 tablespoons of extra virgin olive oil
- ~ 500 g of veal nut
- ~ 30 g of grated Parmesan cheese
- ~ 1 teaspoon of aromas for roasts
- ~ 200 ml (8.8 fl.oz.) dry white wine

Material Required

- ~ Chopping board or pastry board
- ~ Spinach cooking pot
- ~ Cylinder
- ~ Elastic food net
- ~ Casserole with lid
- ~ Scoop
- ~ Grater

Preparation

First, steam the spinach, then let it cool slightly.

Roughly chop the spinach with a knife, then sauté in a pan with salt, pepper, garlic and a dash of extra virgin olive oil.

Open the veal steak and season to taste by adding salt, pepper and roasting herbs. Cover the entire surface with slices of cooked ham, then distribute the chopped spinach. Sprinkle with grated Parmesan cheese.

Gently roll up the roll, starting with the short side.

Insert an elastic food net in the bottom of a cylinder; gently slide the roll into the cylinder, then slide the net along the entire surface of the roll.

Weld the ends of the roll together.

Heat a casserole on the stove: when it is very hot, brown the roll in all its parts.

When browning is complete, pour in plenty of dry white wine and add aromas to taste (sage, rosemary and bay leaves are recommended).

Continue cooking for about an hour and a half, turning the roll from time to time. Meat must always cook in abundant liquid: in case wine evaporates, it is recommended to add more wine or water.

Just before turning off the heat, let any excess liquid dry. Remove the roll from the pan and strain the sauce.

Allow the roll to cool completely before removing the elastic net and cutting.

We recommend cutting the roll into 1 cm thick slices, and accompanying it with the cooking sauce.

Stuffed Turkey Roll

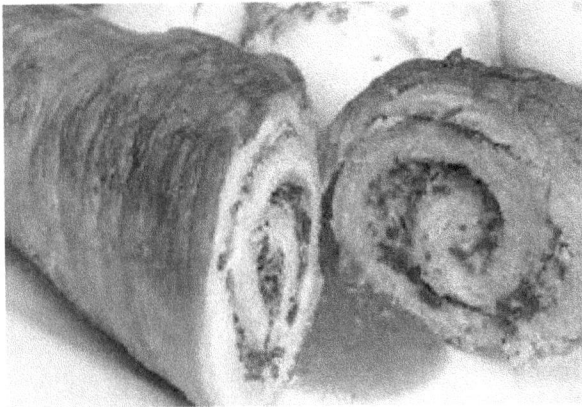

Recipe ID card

- ~ 225 Kcal calories per serving
- ~ Difficult difficulty
- ~ Serves 10
- ~ Preparation 160 minutes
- ~ Average cost
- ~ 2 hours for cooking the cotechino; 40 minutes for cooking the roll

Ingredients

- ~ For the roll
- ~ 1 glass (about 200 ml) of dry white wine
- ~ 400 g of turkey steak
- ~ a few leaves of sage
- ~ salt
- ~ 1 sprig of rosemary
- ~ pepper
- ~ Gluten-free: 500 g of cotechino
- ~ 100 g of carrots
- ~ 1 bay leaf
- ~ 1 garlic clove
- ~ For the side dish
- ~ 1 tablespoon of extra virgin olive oil
- ~ pepper
- ~ salt
- ~ 450 g of carrots

Material Required

- ~ Rigid plastic bottle
- ~ Rolling net
- ~ Latex gloves (optional)
- ~ Tool to remove cores
- ~ Scissors to cut the netting
- ~ Steam cooker
- ~ Casserole with lid for roll
- ~ Pan for cooking carrots
- ~ Cutting board for food
- ~ Pointed stick (toothpick)

Preparation

First, steam the cotechino a couple of hours.

In the meantime prepare the side dish of carrots. After washing and peeling them, cut the carrots into rounds (apart from one, which will be used for stuffing the cotechino) and let them season in a pan with a little oil, salt and pepper. Continue cooking over a gentle flame for 15-20 minutes.

Remove the still hot cotechino from the steam saucepan. Using a knife, cut lengthwise into the surface of the cotechino and remove the casing. It is important to do this while the cotechino is still very hot.

Dig lengthwise the inside of the cotechino with the core lever or with another sharp tool: we should pierce the cotechino in all its length.

Gently push the carrot kept aside inside the cotechino, avoiding that it breaks.

Wrap the cotechino over the turkey steak. Salt the outside to taste. It is not necessary to salt the inside of the roll because the cotechino is already flavorful.

At this point, proceed with shaping the actual roll, pushing it into the mesh as if to form a cage.

Now proceed with the final cooking: brown the roll in a very hot casserole (without adding oil or butter!). When it is well browned, deglaze with white wine and add the aromas: rosemary, sage, bay leaf and garlic.

Continue cooking over low heat for 30-40 minutes.

Let the roll cool down. Using scissors, remove the netting and cut the roll into 1 cm thick slices.

Serve the roll stuffed with cotechino with carrots.

Salmon with Orange Sauce

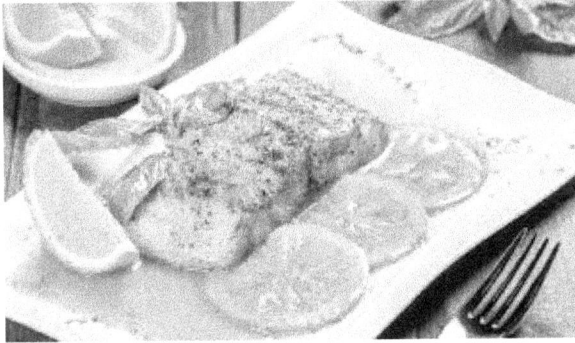

Recipe ID card

~ 77 Kcal calories per serving
~ Easy difficulty
~ Serves 4
~ Preparation 15 minutes
~ Average cost
~ 15 minutes for preparation; 15 minutes for cooking

Ingredients

~ For the salmon
~ 1 slice (600 g) of fresh salmon
~ 50 g of taggiasca or black olives
~ 200 g of fennel
~ 50 ml of dry white wine
~ pepper
~ salt
~ 1 sprig of parsley
~ dill or fennel
~ 1 clove of garlic
~ 600 g (2 large) untreated oranges
~ 1 tablespoon of extra virgin olive oil
~ For the sauce
~ pepper
~ 2 tablespoons of extra virgin olive oil
~ fennel
~ 200 g (1 medium) of untreated oranges
~ 125 g of low-fat yoghurt
~ salt

Material Required

~ Baking sheet
~ Baking paper
~ Bowls of various sizes
~ Row lemons

Preparation

Clean the salmon slice, remove the bones and cut it into regular slices.

Rub a clove of garlic over the salmon. Using a lemon striper, remove the zest from the orange. In a bowl, squeeze the orange juice and emulsify by adding the oil and seasoning with salt, pepper, fennel, parsley and white wine. Peel an orange and remove the pulp.

Preheat the oven to 180°C (ventilated).

Arrange the orange slices on a plate lined with baking paper, then place the salmon slices on top and drizzle with the scented emulsion. Add the Taggiasca olives. Bake the salmon in a hot oven for 12-15 minutes.

Meanwhile, prepare the accompanying sauce by mixing the yoghurt with the orange juice and zest, the fennel, salt, pepper and oil.

Using a knife, cut the fennel into very thin slices, then season to taste with salt, pepper, oil and orange juice.

Remove the salmon from the oven and serve with a fennel salad and yogurt sauce, spreading it over the fish or serving it in a small bowl on the side. If desired, finish with black bread cut into star shapes using steel molds.

Sausage Snake

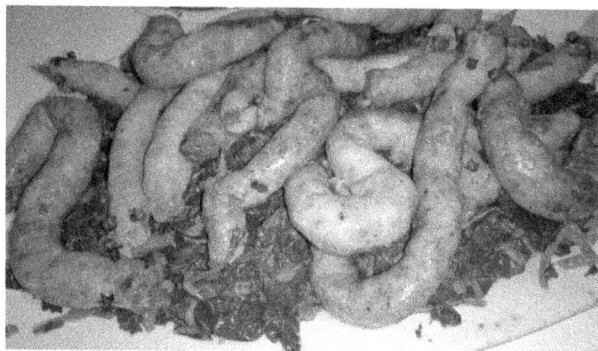

Recipe ID card

- ~ 247 Kcal calories per serving
- ~ Difficulty fairly easy
- ~ Serves 5
- ~ Preparation 20 minutes
- ~ Low cost

Ingredients

- ~ 10 pieces of cloves
- ~ A few pieces of red bell pepper or chili pepper
- ~ 5 pieces (about 250 g) of chicken sausage

To serve

- ~ 150 g of parboiled basmati rice
- ~ A few drops of chlorophyll
- ~ 1 pinch of salt
- ~ 1 drizzle of extra virgin olive oil

Material Required

- ~ Saucepan for cooking rice
- ~ Pasta drainer
- ~ Pan with lid
- ~ 5 long skewer sticks
- ~ Spoon

Preparation

Pour plenty of water into a large saucepan and bring to a boil.

When the water boils, pour in the rice (it is advisable to use a rice that does not shake such as parboiled or basmati) and salt to taste.

Add a few drops of chlorophyll to the cooking water: in this way, the rice will absorb the color and you can get a green rice (with which you will then prepare the "meadow" for the sausage "snakes"). Cook the rice for 12-15 minutes, respecting the cooking time indicated on the package.

In the meantime, prepare the sausage: pierce each chicken sausage with a long skewer stick, trying to obtain a wavy shape that imitates that of the snakes.

If the sticks are too long, cut off the excess.

Brown the sausages well in a very hot pan (without adding oil or butter!), keeping a lively flame. Once the sausages are browned on all sides, cover the pan with the lid, lower the heat to low and continue cooking for a few minutes.

Remove sausages from pan to prevent them from absorbing excess fat. Allow to cool slightly, then gently remove the sticks from the sausages, which will now have taken on a "snake" shape.

Make 2 small holes in one end of each sausage to make the eyes of the snake: simply insert 2 cloves or 2 peppercorns.

For the mouth and tongue, make a horizontal cut under the eyes and insert a small triangular piece of chili bell pepper or red bell pepper.

At this point, the rice will be ready: drain the rice from the water, add a drop of extra virgin olive oil and arrange it on a large serving plate, as if it were a meadow. Place the sausages on top of the green rice and serve.

Vegetable Stew

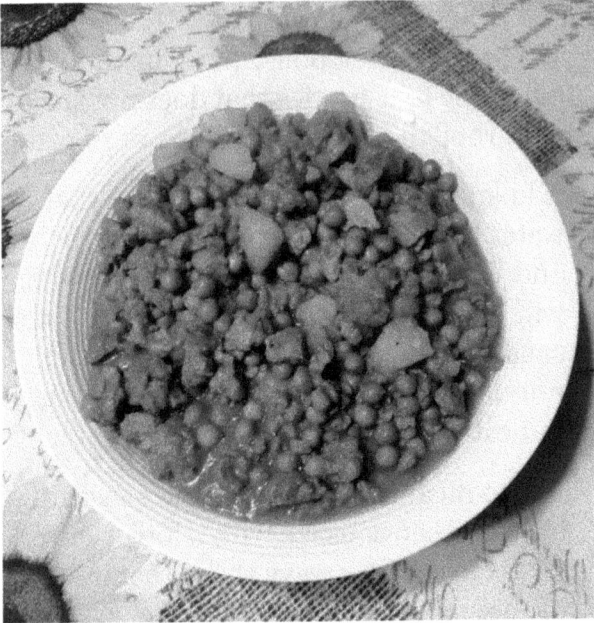

Recipe ID card

- ~ 141 Kcal calories per serving
- ~ Difficulty very easy
- ~ Serves 4
- ~ Preparation 30 minutes
- ~ Low cost

Ingredients

- ~ 1 clove of garlic
- ~ 1 celery stalk
- ~ 1 pinch of salt
- ~ 1 pinch of chilli pepper
- ~ 300 g of tomato puree
- ~ 2 tablespoons of extra virgin olive oil
- ~ 600 g of wheat muscle
- ~ 200 g of carrots
- ~ 1 bay leaf
- ~ 1 teaspoon of brown sugar

Material Required

- ~ Food cutting board
- ~ Saucepan with lid
- ~ Wooden ladle
- ~ Vegetable peeler
- ~ Knife

Preparation

Cut the wheat muscle into fairly regular sized cubes, about the size of a walnut.

Clean the vegetables: wash the carrot, peel it and cut it into rounds. Wash the celery, remove any filaments and cut it into small pieces.

Prepare the tomato sauce. In a casserole, brown the garlic in a little oil and add the tomato puree, celery and carrot cut into rounds. Adjust the salt (we recommend Himalayan pink salt), add the chili pepper, bay leaf and sugar. Cook slowly for 20 minutes.

After this time has elapsed, add the cubes of wheat muscle and let it season for another 10 minutes.

The vegetable stew is ready to serve.

Tuna Slices with Sesame

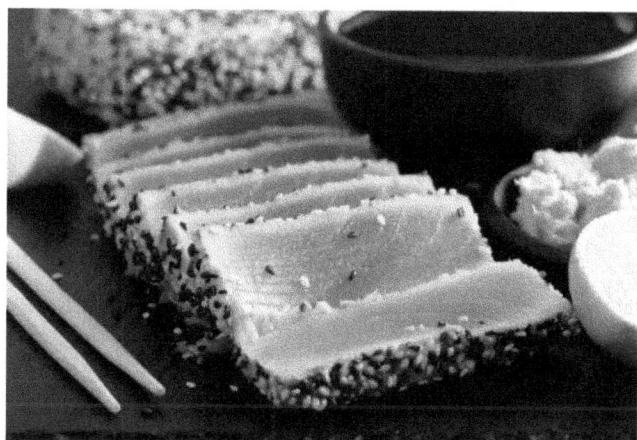

Recipe ID card

~ 176 Kcal calories per serving
~ Difficulty very easy
~ Serves 2
~ Preparation 15 minutes
~ Average cost
~ 10 minutes for preparing and cooking the tuna + 5 minutes for the sauce

Ingredients

~ For the tuna
~ 500 g of fresh tuna
~ about 50 g of sesame seeds
~ 2 tablespoons (20 ml) of extra virgin olive oil
~ Optional: 1 pinch of salt
~ For the sauce
~ 1 pinch of salt
~ 1 tablespoon of extra virgin olive oil
~ 50 g of yoghurt
~ 30 g of almonds
~ 4-5 mint leaves
~ 1 bunch of basil
~ pepper

Material Required

~ Food cutting board
~ Sharp knife
~ Small bowl
~ Stone or non-stick frying pan with lid
~ Immersion mixer
~ High-sided container or beaker

Preparation

Considering how quickly the tuna is cooked, it is advisable to start by preparing the accompanying sauce. In a beaker, pour a few basil and mint leaves (previously washed and dried), the creamy natural yogurt, a tablespoon of extra virgin olive oil, salt, pepper and almonds.

Blend everything with an immersion blender until a thick cream is formed. Those who want an even more fluid sauce can add a couple of tablespoons of yogurt.

Cut the tuna into fairly regular squares, using a very sharp knife.

Dip each cube of tuna in a small bowl full of sesame seeds, applying gentle pressure to facilitate the adhesion of the seeds without damaging the fish.

Heat a stone frying pan and, when very hot, pour in a couple of tablespoons of extra-virgin olive oil.

Cook the tuna steaks covered with seeds in the pan, maintaining a very high flame: for a perfect browning, turn the tuna cubes after 2 minutes only. For "rare" cooking, the tuna should be left in the pan for 3 minutes (about 1.5 minutes per side). It is not necessary to add salt to the tuna because it is a sea fish, already salty by itself.

Serve the tuna cubes hot, accompanied by the mint, almond and basil sauce.

Tripe LIGHT

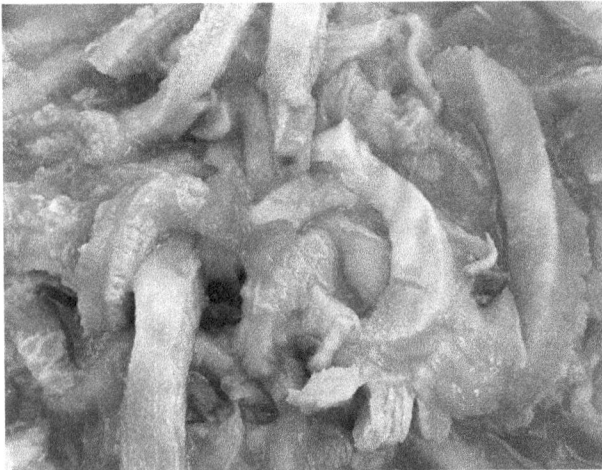

Recipe ID card

- ~ 67 Kcal calories per serving
- ~ Difficulty fairly easy
- ~ Serves 4
- ~ Preparation 30 minutes
- ~ Low cost
- ~ 30 minutes for cleaning; 4 hours for cooking

Ingredients

For the sauce

- ~ 1 teaspoon of tomato concentrate
- ~ 400 ml of broth or dry white wine
- ~ 500-600 g of beef tripe
- ~ 2 celery ribs
- ~ 1 small piece of shallot
- ~ A few leaves of sage
- ~ salt
- ~ 1 sprig of rosemary
- ~ A generous grating of pepper
- ~ 400 g of small pieces of tomato or tomato puree
- ~ 1 berry of juniper
- ~ 1 or 2 pieces of cloves
- ~ 100 g of carrots
- ~ 1 bay leaf
- ~ 1 garlic clove

- ~ 50 ml of vinegar

To serve

- ~ about 30 g of grated Parmesan cheese
- ~ 2 tablespoons of extra virgin olive oil

Material Required

- ~ Ciotole
- ~ Guanti in lattice
- ~ 2 casseruole molto capienti con coperchio
- ~ Schiumarola
- ~ Cucchiaio di legno
- ~ Coltello
- ~ Tagliere
- ~ Garza sterile
- ~ Cordoncino da cucina

Preparation

Wash the tripe in hot running water, rubbing it lightly with your hands. Cut the tripe into 3-4 cm pieces.

In the meantime, bring a saucepan with plenty of water to the boil and add half a glass of vinegar to remove the characteristic organoleptic of the tripe.

Plunge the tripe into the hot water with the vinegar and let it boil for about ten minutes.

Prepare the sauce. Clean the vegetables, then wash the carrots, peel and cut them into small pieces. Wash the celery, remove any hard filaments and cut it into pieces. In a large saucepan, pour the pieces of tomato (or peeled tomatoes), carrots and celery. Then prepare a sterile gauze bag with the mixed spices: in this way, the aromas will not be dispersed in the sauce. In the gauze, add the rosemary, sage, bay leaf, garlic (better if without the heart, which is not easily digested), 1 juniper berry

74

and 1 clove. Close the gauze with a kitchen string and arrange it in the sauce. Then add a small shallot (or half) and a teaspoon of tomato paste. Bring everything to a boil without adding oil.

At this point, remove the tripe from the cooking water with a skimmer, and plunge it into the sauce. Cover with about 2 glasses of dry white wine (or stock) and bring to the boil. Season with salt and add plenty of black pepper. Lower the heat, cover with a lid and cook over very low heat for at least 3-4 hours.

If necessary, add more liquid (wine or broth) during cooking: the tripe should always be well covered with liquid.

When cooked, remove the lid and the bag of aromas and, if necessary, allow the excess liquid to dry, adding only at this point 2 tablespoons of oil. Add the grated grana cheese and mix thoroughly.

Serve the tripe steaming hot, accompanied by rustic bread or slices of polenta.

Eggless and Cholesterol Free Omelette

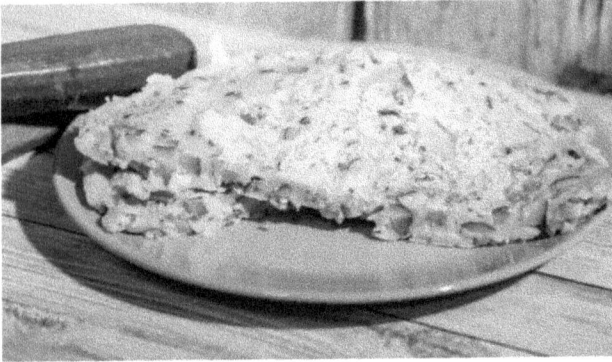

Recipe ID card

~ 103 Kcal calories per serving
~ Easy difficulty
~ Serves 2
~ Preparation 20 minutes
~ Low cost

Ingredients

~ 200 g of chickpea flour
~ 300 ml of water
~ 400 g of zucchini
~ 2 tablespoons of extra virgin olive oil
~ 1 pinch of turmeric
~ 10 g of linseed
~ salt
~ pepper
~ 1 grated nutmeg

Material Required

~ Bowl
~ Whisk
~ 28 cm diameter pan
~ Flat lid
~ Cutting board
~ Knife
~ Sieve

Preparation

First, wash the zucchini and remove the ends. Then dice the zucchini or cut them into very thin slices.

Pour 2 tablespoons of e.v.o. oil into a very hot pan, then brown the diced zucchini over high heat for a couple of minutes. Then lower the heat, add salt and pepper to taste and cook with the lid on for about ten minutes, keeping a gentle flame.

In the meantime, prepare the batter: in a bowl, sift the chickpea flour and add the water, a little at a time, stirring with a whisk until it forms a thick and velvety cream, free of lumps. Season with salt and pepper, spice to taste (e.g. turmeric and nutmeg) and add the flax seeds.

Add the chickpea batter directly into the pan of zucchini, which in the meantime will have become soft: keep a high flame for a couple of minutes, distributing the mixture evenly. Cover with the lid, lower the heat and cook for 7-8 minutes, until the batter has thickened.

Turn the veg-frittata out onto the pan, helping with a flat lid: this will form a golden, inviting crust on both sides of the veg-frittata,

Serve the veg-frittata piping hot.

Sweets and Desserts for Diabetics

Cocoa Diet Bars

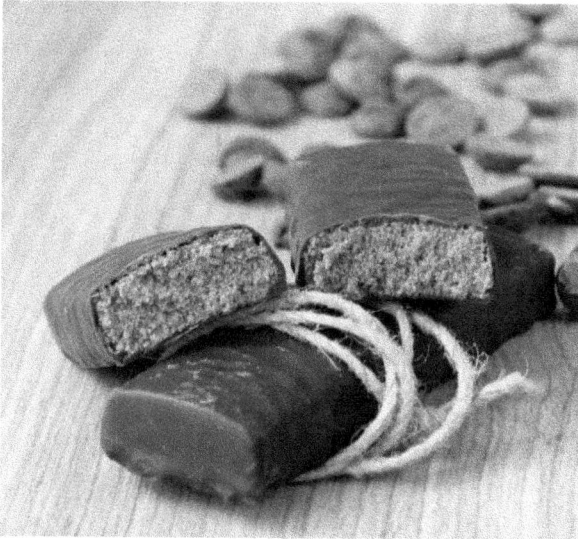

Recipe ID card

- ~ 155 Kcal calories per serving
- ~ Difficulty fairly easy
- ~ Serves 6
- ~ Preparation 25 minutes
- ~ Average cost
- ~ 10 minutes to prepare; 15 minutes to cook + 1 hour to chill

Ingredients

- ~ For the base
- ~ 30 g of wheat bran
- ~ 10 g of whey protein
- ~ 40 g (1 medium) of egg white
- ~ 30 ml of skimmed milk
- ~ 10 g of fructose
- ~ For the filling
- ~ 20 ml skimmed milk
- ~ 3 g of gelatine powder
- ~ 15 g of fructose
- ~ 15 g of bitter cocoa
- ~ 1 grated rind of untreated oranges
- ~ 120 g of low-fat ricotta cheese

Material Required

- ~ Precision scale
- ~ Large bowl
- ~ Wooden spoon
- ~ Baking tray or rectangular mold
- ~ Baking paper
- ~ Long blade knife
- ~ Sieve
- ~ Grater

Preparation

First prepare the base of the bars. In a bowl, mix the wheat bran with the egg white, fructose, protein powder and skimmed milk: you should obtain a firm but easily moldable mixture.

Roll out the dough obtained in a sheet of baking paper, shaping it with a spatula or a knife until obtaining a rectangle with dimensions of 10X20 cm. It is advisable to level the surface of the rectangle with a dampened knife.

Bake the base of the bars in a hot oven at 180°C for 15 minutes. Allow to cool completely.

At this point, prepare the topping of the bars. Warm the milk and dissolve the gelatine powder and fructose in it.

Mix the low-fat ricotta cheese (if possible sieved) with the bitter cocoa powder and the mixture of milk, gelatine and fructose: you should obtain a dense and compact cream.

Pour the cream of ricotta and cocoa on the crunchy base and level with the help of a knife. Let everything rest in the refrigerator for at least an hour, to allow the gelatine to act and congeal.

Remove the cake from the fridge and obtain 6 bars. Grate some orange zest and distribute on the surface of the bars.

Zone diet bars can be stored in the fridge, tightly closed in an airtight container, for 5-7 days.

Vegan Whole Grain Cookies

~ Rolling pin
~ Knife
~ Cutting board
~ Blender

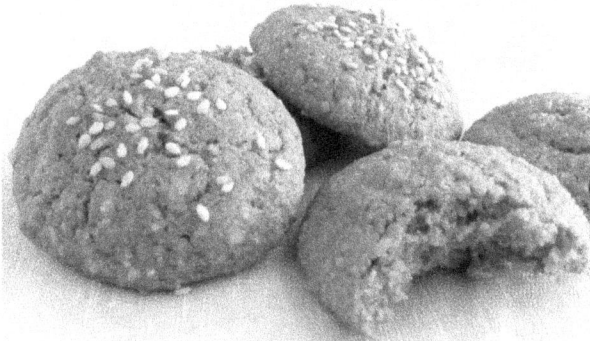

Recipe ID card

~ 319 Kcal calories per serving
~ Easy difficulty
~ Serves 5
~ Preparation 15 minutes
~ Low cost
~ 15 minutes to prepare; 30 minutes to rest; 12-15 minutes to cook

Ingredients for 20 cookies

~ 100 g of wholemeal flour
~ 50 g of oat flakes
~ 40 g of preparation based on stevia and erythritol or another type of sweetener
~ 20 ml of corn seed oil
~ 50 g + 10 g of hazelnuts
~ 50 g of dates
~ 4 g of baking powder
~ 50 ml water
~ 1 pinch of salt

Material Required

~ Food scales
~ Cookie cutters
~ Baking paper
~ Baking tray
~ Wooden spoon

Preparation

In a blender, combine 50 g of hazelnuts and oatmeal: grind until a fine powder is obtained.

Stone the dates, cut them into pieces and combine them in the glass of a blender. Grind the dates until they form a cream.

In a bowl, combine the hazelnut and oat powder, whole-wheat flour, sifted baking powder, salt and stevia and erythritol sweetener.

With your hands, mix the powders with the date cream to form a crumb mixture.

At this point, mix everything with seed oil and water: mix with your hands and obtain a soft and not sticky dough.

Wrap the dough in a sheet of plastic wrap and let rest for half an hour.

Using a rolling pin, roll out the cookie dough on the pastry board, using a little wholemeal flour if necessary. Make a sheet of dough about half an inch thick.

With a cookie cutter shaped as desired get the cookies and place them as you go on a plate lined with baking paper. The scraps can be reshuffled to make more cookies.

Cut the remaining hazelnuts in half.

Insert half a hazelnut in the center of each cookie.

Bake the cookies and bake in a hot oven, preheated to 180°C, for 12 minutes (for soft cookies) or 15 minutes (for crispier cookies).

Remove the cookies from the oven, let them cool and serve.

Vegan cookies with no added sugars can be stored in a tin box for 7-10 days.

Protein Biscuits

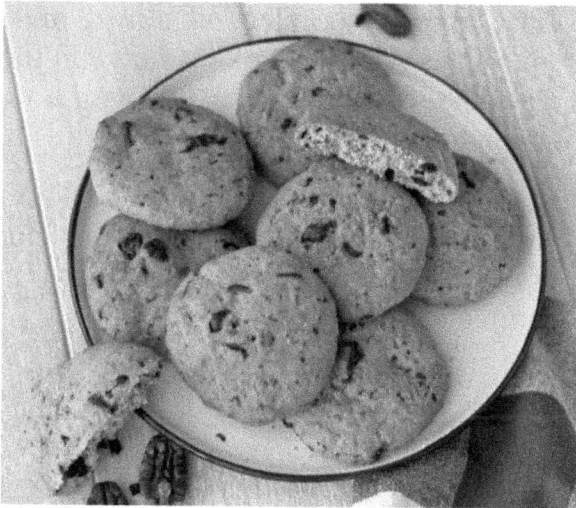

Recipe ID card

- ~ 275 Kcal calories per serving
- ~ Easy difficulty
- ~ Serves 4
- ~ Preparation 21 minutes
- ~ Low cost
- ~ 15 minutes to prepare; 5-6 minutes to cook

Ingredients

- ~ 80 g egg white
- ~ 40 g of peanuts
- ~ 50 g of oat flakes
- ~ 40 g of fructose
- ~ 10 g of inulin
- ~ 5 g of soy lecithin
- ~ 40 g of whey protein

Material Required

- ~ Electric whisk to beat egg whites until stiff
- ~ Sac à poche
- ~ Baking paper
- ~ Leccarda (baking tray)
- ~ Mixer blends everything
- ~ Wooden spoon or pot licker
- ~ Steel spoon

Preparation

First of all, prepare the oat flour starting from the flakes: put the oat flakes in the mixer and blend them finely.

Then prepare the peanuts: after shelling them, blend them in the mixer with the addition of a tablespoon of fructose.

In an electric whisk, whip the two egg whites until stiff. Slowly add the fructose, lowering the speed of the machine to avoid disassembling the egg whites.

Then remove the electric whisk and slowly add all the other ingredients, i.e. the oat flour, finely chopped peanuts, whey protein, inulin and lecithin. Stir with a wooden spoon from the bottom up.

Prepare a drip pan lined with baking paper.

Transfer the foamy mixture obtained in a sac à poche and create many sticks about 8 cm long on the baking paper.

Bake at 180 ° C for 5-6 minutes, ensuring that they do not brown excessively. Wait until the cookies have cooled before removing them from the plate.

Dark chocolate pudding

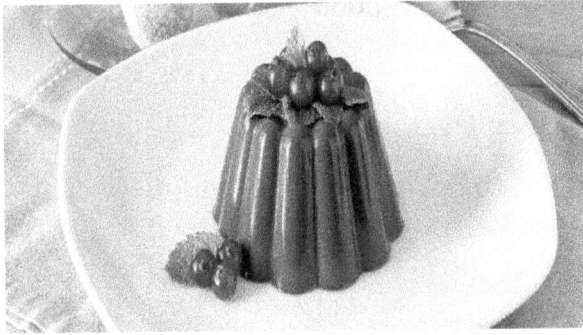

Recipe ID card

- ~ 114 Kcal calories per serving
- ~ Difficulty very easy
- ~ Serves 3
- ~ Preparation 10 minutes
- ~ Low cost
- ~ 10 minutes + cooling time (about 30-40 minutes)

Ingredients 3 puddings

- ~ 300 ml of skimmed milk
- ~ 60 g of dark chocolate
- ~ 30 g of rice flour
- ~ half a small glass of chocolate liqueur or rum
- ~ To decorate (optional)
- ~ dark chocolate chips

Material Required

- ~ Saucepan
- ~ Whisk
- ~ Glass
- ~ Spoon
- ~ 3 pudding molds
- ~ Knife or vegetable peeler for chocolate

Preparation

Heat about 250 ml of skimmed milk in a saucepan. When the milk is hot, add the dark chocolate cut into pieces: stir with a wooden spoon to help it melt.

In the meantime, dissolve the rice flour in the remaining milk, and add it to the saucepan only when the chocolate has melted completely.

Add the rum to the saucepan of milk (alternatively you can add half a small glass of chocolate liqueur).

Stir continuously with the whisk until the mixture has thickened.

Wet the aluminium molds with a little water, then immediately fill them with the hot pudding.

Leave to cool in the refrigerator. Once cold, turn the container out onto a plate: it will be very easy to remove the pudding and it is not necessary to heat the containers with hot water (as you usually do to remove the panna cotta from the mold).

Before serving, decorate with some dark chocolate cut with a vegetable peeler or a sharp knife.

Vanilla Pudding

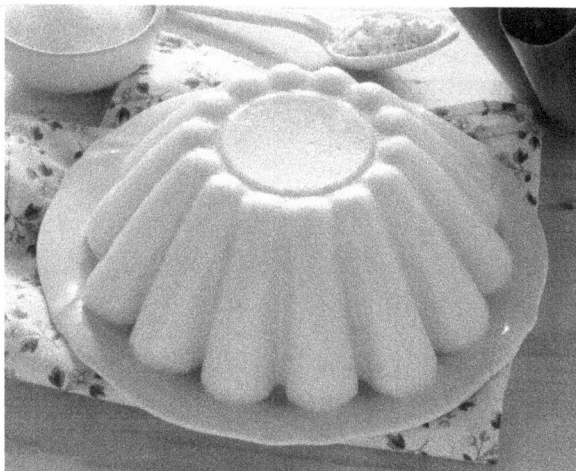

Recipe ID card

~ 113 Kcal calories per serving
~ Easy difficulty
~ Serves 6
~ Preparation 15 minutes
~ Low cost
~ 15 minutes to prepare; 5 minutes to cook; 2 hours to chill

Ingredients

For 6 puddings

~ 550 ml of pasteurized whole milk
~ 18 g of preparation based on sodium saccharin, sorbitol, mannitol, fructose or another type of sweetener
~ 6 g of isinglass
~ 30 g of cornstarch
~ 1 vanilla pod

For the sauce

~ 50 g of dark chocolate
~ 2 g of preparation based on sodium saccharin, sorbitol, mannitol, fructose or another type of sweetener
~ 1 tablespoon of corn seed oil

Material Required

~ Food scale
~ Casserole
~ Whisk
~ Silicone molds
~ Colander

Preparation

First, soak the isinglass sheets so that they soften.

Cut into a vanilla pod and scrape out the seeds with the tip of a knife.

In a small saucepan, pour about 400 ml of whole milk and flavor with the vanilla seeds and the pod. Heat for 5 minutes over low heat.

In a bowl, pour the remaining cold milk and, with a whisk, dissolve the corn-starch in it.

Strain the hot milk to remove any strands released from the pod.

Bring the vanilla milk back to the heat and add the sweetener and starch dissolved in the cold milk. Bring to a boil taking care to maintain a gentle flame. Turn off the heat and add the sheets of isinglass, well squeezed out of the soaking water.

Distribute the pudding in single-portion moulds and leave to cool in the fridge for at least two hours. To speed up the firming of the pudding and make it easier to remove from the mold, we recommend freezing.

Meanwhile, prepare the chocolate sauce. Chop the dark chocolate and melt it gently in the microwave or in a bain-marie. Add the sweetener and a tablespoon of seed oil. Mix the mixture until shiny and glossy.

Turn the puddings out of the molds by gently inverting them onto individual plates and decorate with chocolate sauce.

Budino Antiage and Antiosidante

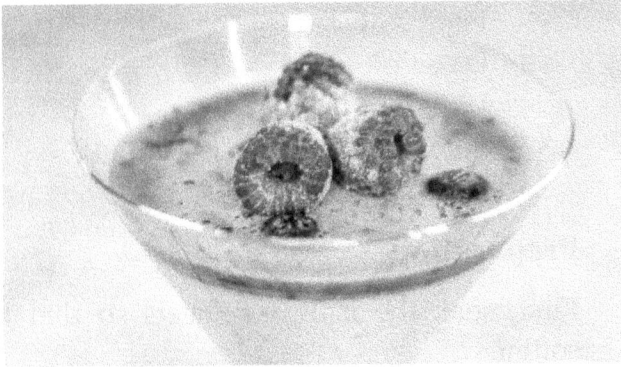

Recipe ID card

~ Difficulty quite easy
~ Serves 3
~ Preparation 20 minutes
~ Average cost
~ 20 minutes to prepare; 4 hours to chill

Ingredients

For the Raspberry Pudding

~ 150 ml of milk
~ 100 g of yogurt
~ 5 g of isinglass
~ 10 g of stevia
~ 75 g of raspberries

For the blueberry topping

~ 75 g of blueberries
~ 100 ml water
~ 4 g of stevia
~ 2.5 g isinglass

Material Required

~ Glasses or cups
~ Food scale
~ Immersion mixer
~ Colander

Preparation

First, soak the isinglass in cold water.

Pour the milk into a small saucepan and bring to the boil.

Pour the yogurt and raspberries into a beaker, then blend with an immersion blender. If desired, strain the yogurt smoothie through a sieve to remove the seeds.

When the milk is hot, add the stevia and the isinglass, now softened. Mix the mixture with the raspberry yogurt and distribute over 3 cups, up to half the capacity.

Let cool completely for a couple of hours.

When the pudding has firmed up, prepare the second part. Soak the remaining isinglass sheets in cold water. Blend one part blueberries with 80 ml water and stevia. Heat the remaining 20 ml water and dissolve the isinglass in it. Add the isinglass to the blueberry mixture and distribute over the raspberry puddings.

Allow the pudding to set again in the fridge for a couple of hours.

The anti-aging and antioxidant pudding has a consistency similar to aspic: it will keep in the fridge for 3-4 days.

Pudding with Strawberries and Yogurt

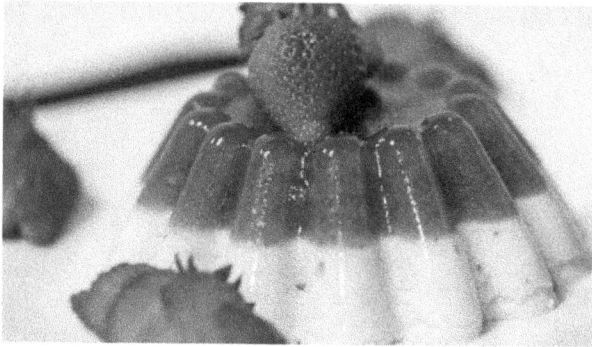

Recipe ID card

~ 35 Kcal calories per serving
~ Easy difficulty
~ Serves 2
~ Preparation 140 minutes
~ Low cost
~ 20 minutes to prepare + 2 hours to chill

Ingredients

For the strawberry base

~ 150 g of strawberries
~ untreated lemon juice
~ 40 g of erythritol
~ 4 g (2 sheets) of isinglass

For the yoghurt base

~ 2 tablespoons of water
~ 4 g (2 sheets) of isinglass
~ 20 g of erythritol
~ 70 g of strawberries
~ 150 g of yoghurt

Material Required

~ Silicone mold 400 ml
~ Saucepan
~ Immersion mixer with container
~ Wooden ladle
~ Bowls of various sizes
~ Ceramic knives
~ Cutting board for food

Preparation

Soak two sheets of isinglass in a small bowl filled with cold water.

In the meantime, wash the strawberries thoroughly, removing the non-edible parts; then dry them well, cut them into small pieces and pour them into a high-sided container. Add the erythritol and the filtered juice of half a lemon (very useful to avoid oxidation of the strawberries).

Pour the strawberries with the erythritol and lemon juice into a small pan and heat the mixture slightly. Add the soaked and well squeezed isinglass, stirring gently until the thickener is completely dissolved.

Pour the liquid obtained into a silicone mold, filling it up to half.

Place the mold in the refrigerator to cool and solidify.

Proceed with the preparation of the second layer. Wash the remaining strawberries (70 g) and blend them with the erythritol. Pour in the yoghurt and stir with a wooden spoon to mix the mixture.

Soak the 2 sheets of isinglass in cold water.

Heat a couple of tablespoons of water in a small pan, then add the softened and well squeezed isinglass. Pour the mixture into the yogurt cream and mix.

Spread the yogurt cream over the first layer of strawberries, which in the meantime will have solidified perfectly.

Put the mold back in the refrigerator for a couple of hours or so, to allow the isinglass to thicken everything.

Turn the mold out onto a serving plate, decorate the pudding as desired with fresh strawberries and serve.

Vanilla Soy Pudding

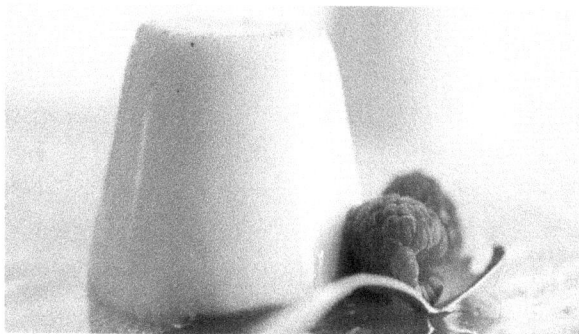

Recipe ID card

- ~ 72 Kcal calories per serving
- ~ Easy difficulty
- ~ Serves 2
- ~ Preparation 10 minutes
- ~ Average cost
- ~ 10 minutes + cooling time (about 30 minutes)

Ingredients

For two puddings

- ~ 200 ml soy milk
- ~ 10 g of soy flour
- ~ 20 g of fructose
- ~ 2 g of agar
- ~ 1 stick or 1 vanilla pod

For the sauce (optional)

- ~ 150 g of peaches
- ~ 1 tablespoon of fructose
- ~ half a small glass of untreated lemon juice

Material Required

- ~ 2 aluminum molds (capacity: 100 ml)
- ~ Saucepan
- ~ Whisk
- ~ Frying pan
- ~ Serving dish
- ~ Colander
- ~ Food thermometer

Preparation

In a saucepan pour the soy milk (better if self-produced) and fructose: heat the mixture and add, under constant agitation and very slowly, the soy flour.

Continue to stir with the whisk: a thin layer of foam will begin to form. When it reaches 80°C, add the agar agar, without stopping stirring.

Remove the saucepan from the heat and add the vanilla flavor.

Distribute the mixture into two pudding molds, possibly straining the mixture through a sieve to remove excess foam.

Allow the puddings to cool, first at room temperature, then in the refrigerator, so that they can set perfectly.

Prepare the accompanying sauce: wash, dry and cut the peach into pieces. Fry the peach with the fructose and lemon juice. Those who wish can also flavor the peach with a few drops of vanilla. Allow to cook over gentle heat until the desired consistency is reached.

To remove the pudding from the mold, simply dip the container in boiling water for a few moments and immediately invert it onto a serving plate.

Serve by accompanying the pudding with the peach sauce.

Strawberry tart for diabetics

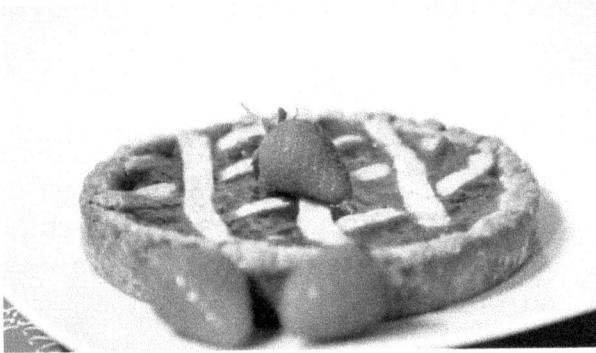

Recipe ID card

~ 179 Kcal calories per serving
~ Easy difficulty
~ Serves 6
~ Preparation 40 minutes
~ Average cost
~ 20 minutes for the preparation of the tart + the baking time (about 20 minutes)

Ingredients

For the shortcrust pastry (for a baking pan with a diameter of 18 cm)

~ 1 pinch of salt
~ 1 sachet of vanillin
~ 60 g (1 medium) of eggs
~ 35 ml of corn seed oil
~ 10 g of inulin
~ 20 g of fructose
~ 70 g of wholemeal flour
~ 75 g of white flour type 00
~ 20 g of erythritol

For the filling

~ 15 ml of untreated lemon juice
~ 25 g of erythritol
~ 250 g of strawberries

Material Required

~ Large bowl
~ Smaller bowl for steeping strawberries
~ Pastry board
~ Transparent film
~ Hinged baking pan with a diameter of 18 cm
~ Small frying pan for cooking strawberries
~ Baking paper
~ Strawberry knife
~ Ladles

Preparation

First, wash the strawberries and gently dry them with paper towels. Remove the non-edible parts and reduce them into small pieces. Pour the strawberries into a bowl, add the filtered lemon juice and the erythritol: let the strawberries macerate for about twenty minutes.

Meanwhile, prepare the shortcrust pastry. Pour into a bowl the "dry" ingredients, that is the two flours (white and wholemeal flour), the salt, the fructose, the erythritol, the inulin and the vanillin. Mix thoroughly.

Now add the seed oil and the egg: mix first with a wooden spoon, then with hands until a smooth, homogeneous and elastic ball is obtained: the consistency of the dough must be that of a classic shortcrust pastry.

Wrap the dough on a sheet of plastic wrap and let the dough rest in the refrigerator for about twenty minutes: in this way, it will be easier to roll out the pastry with a rolling pin.

While the dough is resting in the fridge, prepare the filling. Pour the strawberries (with the sauce that has formed) into a small pan and cook for about ten minutes, stirring often to prevent the mixture from sticking to the bottom of the pan. Leave the sauce in the pan to cool.

Line an 18 cm diameter hinged baking pan with baking paper.

Remove the shortcrust pastry from the fridge and roll it out on a well-floured pastry board. Spread the pastry in the cake tin, leaving a high border to hold the filling.

Pour the "strawberry jam" directly on top of the shortcrust pastry and decorate, if necessary, with small balls of dough.

Bake in a hot oven (180°C) for about 20 minutes.

Cake with fructose

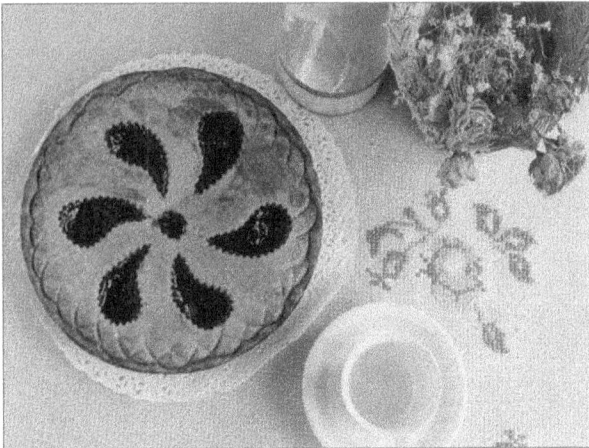

Recipe ID card

~ 283 Kcal calories per serving
~ Easy difficulty
~ Serves 8
~ Preparation 45 minutes
~ Low cost
~ 10 minutes to prepare dough; 5 minutes to peel apples; 30 minutes

Ingredients

~ 350g of white flour type 00
~ 300 g (2 large) apples
~ 150 g of apple jam
~ half a small glass of rum
~ 8 g (half a sachet) of baking powder
~ 30 ml (2 tablespoons, if necessary) of milk
~ 90 g of fructose
~ 80 g (4 medium) egg yolks
~ 150 g butter
~ untreated lemon juice

Material Required

~ 2 large boules (bowls)
~ 1 rolling pin
~ 1 wooden spoon
~ baking paper
~ 1 baking pan with a diameter of 28 cm
~ 1 sieve to filter the lemon juice

Preparation

First, separate the yolks from the egg whites: in a large boule mix the 4 yolks with the room temperature butter (or melted in the microwave) and the fructose.

Mix with a whisk until the mixture is smooth and foamy. Then add the rum, sifted flour and baking powder: if the mixture is too hard to mix with a wooden spoon, add two tablespoons of milk.

When the ingredients are well amalgamated, transfer the shortcrust pastry on the working surface and mix energetically and firmly for a couple of minutes.

Let the dough rest for half an hour.

Meanwhile, wash and peel a couple of large Golden apples. Proceed by cutting them into thin slices and transfer them into a large bowl with the juice of half a lemon, which is essential to prevent oxidation of the apples.

After half an hour, roll out the shortcrust pastry with the help of a rolling pin until it reaches a thickness of about 0.5 cm.

Line a baking pan with baking paper and carefully roll out the pastry inside, ending with a small raised edge to prevent the filling from leaking out of the pastry.

Proceed by adding three spoonfuls of light apple jam directly onto the surface of the pastry, and complete by arranging the apples in a neat radial pattern.

If you wish, you can brush the apples with a bit of apple jam, made more liquid by adding a couple of tablespoons of water (essential to facilitate the drafting with a brush): this small and easy trick will make the apples much brighter.

Bake the cake in a hot oven for 30-35 minutes.

Grandma's Cake without butter

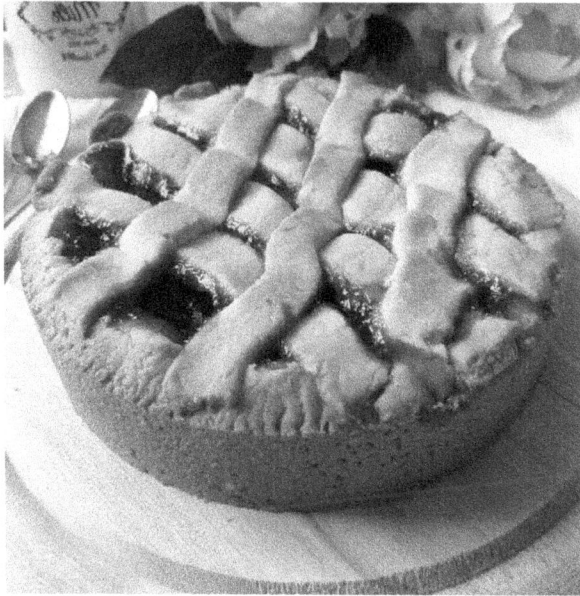

Recipe ID card

~ 219 Kcal calories per serving
~ Easy difficulty
~ Serves 8
~ Preparation 230 minutes
~ Low cost
~ 10 minutes to prepare the shortcrust pastry + 3 hours' rest in the refrigerator; 10 minutes for the light custard; 30 minutes to bake the tart.

Ingredients

For the shortcrust pastry without butter (about 500 g)

~ 60 g (1 medium) eggs
~ 20 ml milk
~ 15 ml of rum
~ 270 g white flour type 00
~ 8 g of baking powder
~ 50 ml of corn oil
~ 40 g of fructose
~ 20 g (1 medium) of egg yolks

To decorate

~ 30 g of pine nuts

For the light custard

~ 4 g of guar gum
~ 1 small vial of lemon flavouring
~ 20 g of potato starch
~ 40 g of fructose
~ 40 g (2 medium) egg yolks
~ 500 ml of soy milk

Material Required

~ Large bowl
~ Baking sheet with a diameter of 26 cm
~ Baking paper
~ Matter
~ Wooden ladles
~ Custard pot
~ Whisk
~ Electric whisk for the custard

Preparation

Preparing the shortcrust pastry without butter is very simple and fast: in a large bowl pour the white flour, fructose, salt, sifted baking powder and mix well.

Add the whole egg, the yolk, the rum, the milk and the oil: mix all the ingredients, first with a wooden spoon, then with your hands, until you get a smooth and soft dough.

Let the shortcrust pastry rest for at least three hours in the refrigerator, to give the cake a better crumbliness.

At this point, prepare the light custard (we recommend referring to the video dedicated to the preparation).

Roll out the shortcrust pastry without butter with a rolling pin until it reaches a thickness of 6-7 mm. Line a cake pan with a diameter of 26 cm with baking paper, then cover with the shortcrust pastry leaving a thick border, which can contain the cream.

Pour the light custard over the shortcrust pastry, until it covers the whole surface of the cake. Finish with a few pine nuts and place the cake in a hot oven at 180°C for 35 minutes.

Leave to cool and serve, decorating if desired.

Ricotta Tart

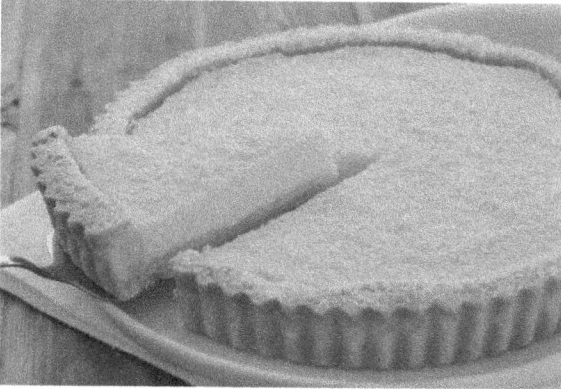

Recipe ID card

- ~ 296 Kcal calories per serving
- ~ Easy difficulty
- ~ Serves 8
- ~ Preparation 45 minutes
- ~ Average cost
- ~ 10 minutes to prepare the shortcrust; 5 minutes to make the cream; 30 minutes to bake.

Ingredients

For the shortcrust pastry

- ~ 350 g of white flour type 00
- ~ 2 tablespoons (30 ml, if necessary) of milk
- ~ 8 g (half a sachet) of baking powder
- ~ grated rind of untreated lemon
- ~ 140 g of butter
- ~ 150 g of sugar
- ~ 80 g (4 medium) egg yolks

For the cream

- ~ 150 g of raisins
- ~ 60 g (one medium) of eggs
- ~ 300 g of fresh ricotta
- ~ half a small glass of rum
- ~ 20 g of pine nuts
- ~ water
- ~ 120 g of sugar

Material Required

- ~ 2 large bowls
- ~ 1 rolling pin
- ~ 1 wooden spoon
- ~ baking paper
- ~ 1 baking pan with a diameter of 26 cm
- ~ Small knife to grate the lemon rind
- ~ 1 electric blender for the cream (optional)
- ~ 1 colander
- ~ 1 honeycomb mold or cookie cutters

Preparation

The first thing to do is to prepare the shortcrust pastry. In a large bowl, pour the flour, add the sugar, butter at room temperature or melted in the microwave, egg yolks and sifted baking powder. Finish by grating the zest of an untreated lemon to make it smell nice.

Mix with a wooden spoon to amalgamate the ingredients. In case the mixture is too hard to mix with the wooden spoon, add a couple of tablespoons of milk.

Pour the mixture on a pastry board and mix until the dough is smooth and homogeneous. Let the dough rest for half an hour.

Meanwhile, prepare the ricotta cream. First, soak the raisins in boiling water and rum for a few minutes.

In an electric whisk, pour the sugar, egg and ricotta: mix at moderate speed for a couple of minutes.

Add the well squeezed raisins and pine nuts to the ricotta mixture and mix with a wooden spoon.

Using a rolling pin, roll out the shortcrust pastry on a sheet of baking paper, making sure not to make it too thin. Transfer the mixture into a baking pan (hinged ones are recommended) with a diameter of 26 cm.

At this point, pour the ricotta mixture over the shortcrust pastry.

Decorate as desired with scraps of shortcrust pastry. Alternatively, create a honeycomb "lid" with the appropriate tool: in this way, the cake will look like it was prepared by a pastry chef!

Bake the cake in a lowered oven, preheated to 180°C, for about 25-30 minutes.

Strawberry ice cream

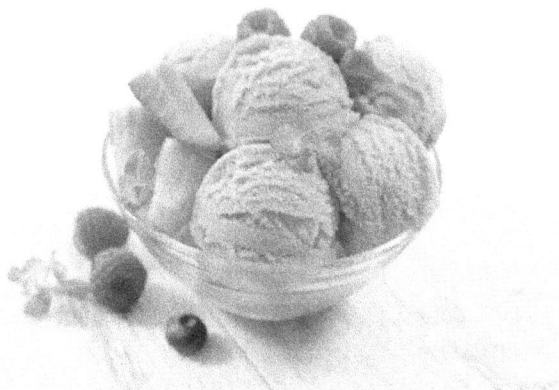

Recipe ID card

~ 46 Kcal calories per serving
~ Difficulty very easy
~ Serves 6
~ Preparation 40 minutes
~ Low cost
~ 10 minutes to prepare; about 30 minutes to freeze in the ice cream maker + time to cool the ice cream maker

Ingredients

~ 350 g of strawberries
~ 500 ml of semi-skimmed milk
~ 60-80 of fructose
~ 20 g of inulin

Material Required

~ Ice cream maker
~ Immersion mixer
~ Jug or container with high sides
~ Wooden ladle
~ Ceramic knife
~ Chopping board

Preparation

Wash the strawberries quickly with fresh water and dry them well so that they do not absorb too much liquid.

Remove the non-edible parts with a ceramic knife and cut them into more or less regular pieces.

Pour the strawberries into a pitcher or another container with high sides, add 60-80 g of fructose and mix with a wooden spoon.

Then pour in the semi-skimmed milk and inulin. Blend everything with an immersion blender until it forms a rather thick liquid.

Transfer the mixture into an ice cream maker and let the ice cream churn for about 20-30 minutes, until the desired consistency is obtained.

Serve the ice-cream in small cups, decorating with a strawberry to taste.

Homemade Kefir

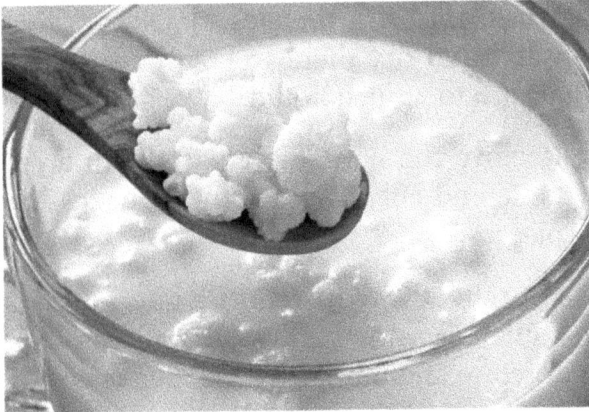

Recipe ID card

- ~ 60 Kcal calories per serving
- ~ Difficulty fairly easy
- ~ Serves 7
- ~ Preparation 15 minutes
- ~ Average cost
- ~ 15 minutes to prepare; 4 hours rest in the yogurt maker; 24 hours rest at room temperature

Ingredients

To prepare 7 jars of Kefir

- ~ 1 L of vegetable milk (rice, soy, almond, coconut), or 1 L of goat's milk, or 1 L of sheep's milk, or 1 L of pasteurized whole milk
- ~ 1 sachet of kefir starter

Material Required

- ~ Cooker
- ~ Food thermometer
- ~ Yogurt maker or thermos
- ~ Glass jars with respective caps
- ~ Wooden spoon
- ~ Ladle (if necessary)

Preparation

Pour milk (any kind of animal or vegetable milk) in a saucepan and heat until it reaches 42°C (42°F).

Pour the mixture of bacteria and yeasts for kefir in a glass and add a part of milk (about 100 ml) until it is completely dissolved.

Add the mixture of microorganisms to the remaining milk and mix thoroughly for a couple of minutes.

Distribute the milk with yeasts and bacteria in single-dose glasses/jars and let it rest for 4-6 hours in a yoghurt maker or pour it in a thermos.

After this time, remove the jars from the yoghurt maker (or thermos) and let it rest at room temperature (24°C) for 20-24 hours.

At the end of 24 hours, kefir is ready to be tasted and can be kept in the fridge for 7-10 days. Individual jars of kefir can be used as a starter to make more kefir.

Cocoa Muffins without Butter

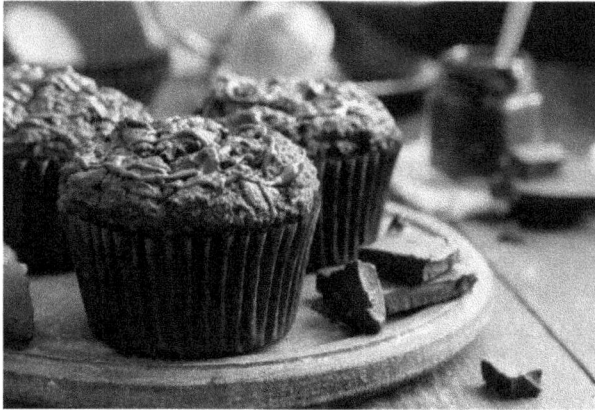

Recipe ID card

- ~ 198 Kcal calories per serving
- ~ Difficulty fairly easy
- ~ Serves 5
- ~ Preparation 25 minutes
- ~ Low cost
- ~ 10 minutes for preparation + 15 minutes for cooking

Ingredients

For 10-12 muffins

- ~ 250 g of fresh ricotta
- ~ 70 g of cornstarch
- ~ 60 g of fructose
- ~ 180 g (3 medium) eggs
- ~ 1 pinch of salt
- ~ 8 g of baking powder
- ~ 15 g of bitter cocoa

Material Required

- ~ Muffin tins
- ~ Muffin mold
- ~ Large bowl
- ~ Electric whisk
- ~ Precision scales
- ~ Sieve
- ~ Spatula
- ~ Ladle

Preparation

In the container of an electric beater, cream the eggs with the fructose. Add the ricotta and salt.

In a bowl, sift the unsweetened cocoa and the yeast, add the corn-starch then gradually add the powders to the eggs and fructose mixture, continuing to mix.

Preheat oven to 180°C.

Insert the muffin cups in the mould, then fill the single-dose containers up to ¾ of their capacity with the cocoa mixture (using a ladle with a measuring spout). You will obtain 10-12 muffins.

Bake the mold at 180°C and bake for 15 minutes. Turn off the oven and let the muffins rest 5 minutes before removing them. For "soft hearted" muffins, bake for 12 minutes and immediately remove the mold from the oven.

Serve the muffins cold.

Dukan Diet Muffins

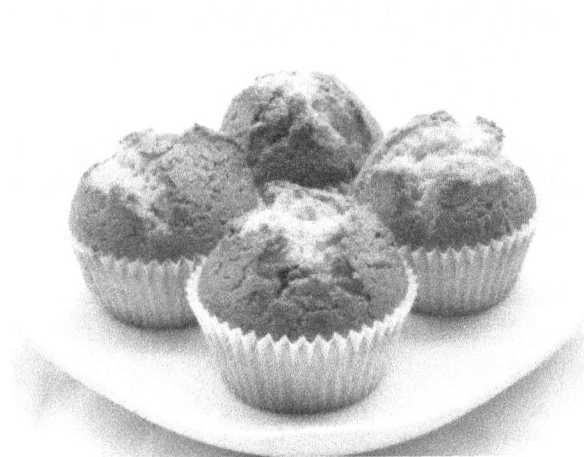

Recipe ID card

- ~ 202 Kcal calories per serving
- ~ Difficulty fairly easy
- ~ Serves 6
- ~ Preparation 25 minutes
- ~ Average cost
- ~ 10 minutes for preparation + 15 minutes for cooking

Ingredients

- ~ 10 tablespoons (150 g) oat bran
- ~ 4 tablespoons (120 g) of low-fat ricotta cheese
- ~ 20 drops of TIC sweetener or sucralose or 100 g of erythritol
- ~ 80 g (4 medium) egg yolks
- ~ 160 g (4 medium) egg whites
- ~ 1 vial of vanilla flavor
- ~ 1 teaspoon of baking powder
- ~ 1 pinch of salt

Material Required

- ~ Bowl
- ~ Wooden spoon
- ~ Electric whisk
- ~ Paper or silicone ramekins
- ~ Muffin mold
- ~ Spatula
- ~ Sieve

Preparation

Preheat the oven to 180°C.

Peel the eggs and separate the whites from the yolks. Whip the egg whites until stiff, adding a pinch of salt.

Meanwhile, mix the oat bran with the erythritol, vanilla flavor, sifted baking powder, low-fat ricotta cheese and yolks. Mix well until the mixture is creamy and thick.

Gradually stir in the stiffly beaten egg whites from the bottom upwards until the mixture is smooth and free of lumps.

Place the paper or silicone cups in the muffin molds provided. Fill each mold with the cream obtained, up to half a centimeter from the edge.

Put the mould in a hot oven (180°C) and bake for 15 minutes. Before removing the mold, let the muffins rest 10 minutes in the oven off; then remove the mold and take out the muffins.

Dukan muffins will keep in an airtight container or nylon bag for up to a week.

Apple Pie Without Added Sugars

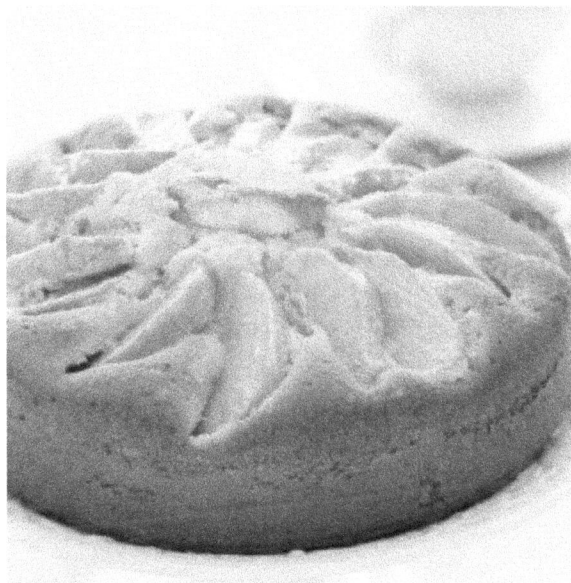

Recipe ID card

~ 154 Kcal calories per serving
~ Easy difficulty
~ Serves 8
~ Preparation 20 minutes
~ Low cost
~ 20 minutes for preparation; 40 minutes for cooking

Ingredients

For the dough

~ 600 g apples
~ 10 g of baking powder
~ 60 ml of corn oil
~ 1 pinch of salt
~ 1 pinch of cinnamon
~ 150 ml of milk
~ 20 g of pine nuts
~ 100 g of raisins
~ Untreated lemon juice and zest
~ 100 g of wholemeal flour
~ 100 g of white flour type 00
~ 50 g of stevia and erythritol or another type of sweetener

~ 60 g (1 medium) of eggs

For the covering

~ 20 g of yellow corn flour
~ 200 g of apples
~ 10 g stevia and erythritol or other sweetener

Material Required

~ Bowl
~ Cutting board
~ Vegetable peeler
~ Sieve
~ Knife
~ Grater or lemon line
~ Baking paper
~ Square baking pan with a side of 22 cm

Preparation

First, soften the raisins in warm water.

Peel the apples, cut them into four parts and remove the stem. Then cut the apple pulp into small cubes. As you get the dicing done, drizzle the apples with lemon juice to prevent rapid oxidation.

In a frying pan, toast the pine nuts for 2-3 minutes: this way, they will become more aromatic.

Preheat the oven to 200°C (static).

Drain the raisins from their soaking water.

In a bowl, combine the white flour and whole wheat flour. Add the diced apple, toasted pine nuts, squeezed raisins and grated lemon zest. Flavor with a teaspoon of cinnamon powder, add a pinch of salt and sweeten with the stevia and erythritol sweetener.

Sift the baking powder and add it to the rest of the ingredients.

Add the egg, seed oil and milk, then mix all ingredients together to form a batter.

Line a 22 cm square baking pan with baking paper. Pour the batter into the pan.

Peel the remaining apple and cut it into thin slices. Embed the apple slices on the surface of the dough, finish with a teaspoon of sweetener and a teaspoon of cornmeal (for gratin).

Bake the cake at 200°C for about 40 minutes, or until the surface is golden brown.

Remove the cake from the oven, let cool, cut into slices and serve.

Pear Cake for Diabetics

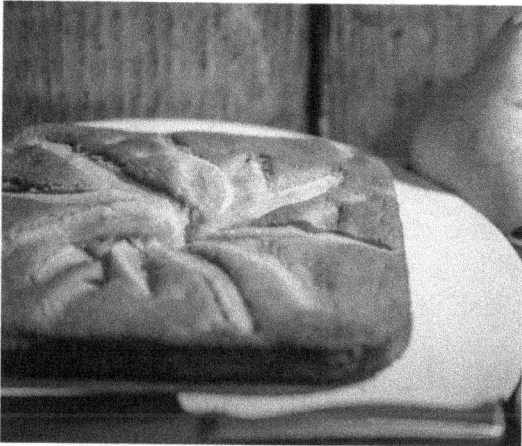

Recipe ID card

- ~ 139 Kcal calories per serving
- ~ Easy difficulty
- ~ Serves 4
- ~ Preparation 20 minutes
- ~ Average cost
- ~ 20 minutes for preparation; 40 minutes for cooking

Ingredients

- ~ 600 g of pears
- ~ 60 g (1 medium) of eggs
- ~ 70 g of erythritol
- ~ 60 ml of corn oil
- ~ 100 ml of skimmed milk
- ~ Wholemeal product: 150 g spelt flour
- ~ 10 g of baking powder
- ~ 30 g of oat bran
- ~ 1 pinch of cinnamon

Material Required

- ~ Square baking pan with a side of 22 cm
- ~ Bowl
- ~ Immersion mixer
- ~ Food scale
- ~ Chopping board
- ~ Knife
- ~ Sieve

Preparation

Peel the pears and cut them into pieces, leaving some slices whole for decoration.

Pour half the pear pulp into a beaker, add the milk and the egg. Blend everything with an immersion blender until you get a liquid cream.

In a bowl, mix the whole wheat spelt flour, bran, erythritol, sifted baking powder and cinnamon.

In the center, pour the obtained shake and the oil. Mix all the ingredients together until a batter is obtained.

At this point, add the remaining pear pieces. Pour the batter into a square baking pan lined with baking paper and decorate the center with the whole pear slices.

Put the cake in the oven and bake at 180°C for 40 minutes. During baking the cake will not swell a lot, but it will still be very soft and fluffy.

Allow to cool, remove from the baking paper and serve in cubes.

Lemon wholemeal cake

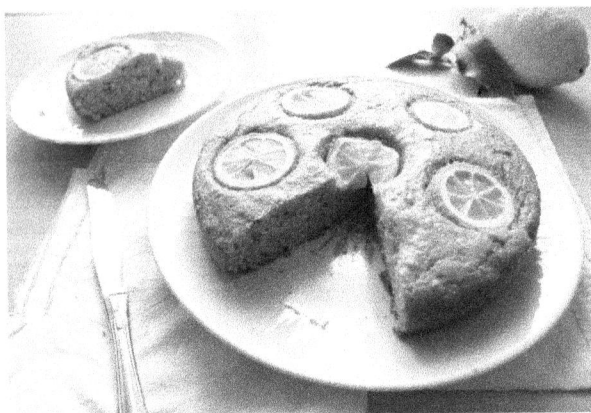

Recipe ID card

- ~ 347 Kcal calories per serving
- ~ Difficulty very easy
- ~ Serves 6
- ~ Preparation 40 minutes
- ~ Low cost
- ~ 10 minutes to prepare; 30 minutes to cook

Ingredients

- ~ 130 g of whole wheat flour
- ~ 120 g (2 medium) eggs
- ~ 90 ml of corn seed oil
- ~ 16 g (1 sachet) of baking powder
- ~ 20 g of stevia
- ~ juice and grated rind of untreated lemon
- ~ 1 small vial of lemon flavouring

Material Required

- ~ Glass or plastic bowl
- ~ Steel or plastic container for the main dough
- ~ Electric whisk
- ~ Spatula pan licker
- ~ Hinged baking pan with a diameter of 18 cm
- ~ Baking paper
- ~ Narrow-mesh sieve
- ~ Lemon zest grater

Preparation

Peel the eggs and separate the yolks from the whites: whip the whites until stiff, adding a pinch of salt if necessary.

Pour the yolks and the stevia into another container, grate the rind of a large untreated lemon and add the juice, filtered through a fine-mesh strainer. Operate the electric whips and mix for a few minutes.

At this point, add the whole-wheat flour, sifted baking powder, oil and lemon flavor. Mix for a few minutes with the electric whips: you should obtain a rather dense mixture.

Finally, add slowly and a little at a time the egg whites whipped to stiff peaks.

Line a hinged baking pan with a diameter of 18 cm with baking paper, then pour the mixture obtained.

Bake in a ventilated oven, preheated to 180°C, and continue cooking for 30-35 minutes.

Leave the cake to cool on a grating and serve, accompanying the cake with a few slices of lemon.

Rustic Pumpkin Pie

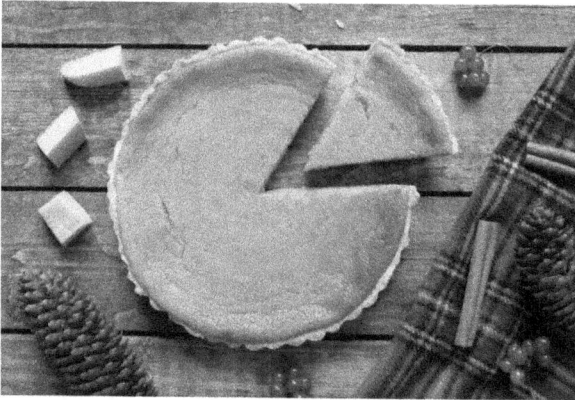

Recipe ID card

- ~ 118 Kcal calories per serving
- ~ Difficult difficulty
- ~ Serves 8
- ~ Preparation 70 minutes
- ~ Average cost
- ~ 30 minutes to prepare + 40 minutes to cook

Ingredients

For the dough

- ~ 550 g of pumpkin pulp
- ~ 150 g of raisins
- ~ 1 pinch of salt
- ~ 2 tablespoons of extra virgin olive oil
- ~ 150 g (1 medium) of apples
- ~ 1 sachet of baking powder
- ~ 150 g of wholemeal flour

For the topping

- ~ 100 ml water
- ~ 50 g of brown sugar
- ~ 300 g apples

Material Required

- ~ Food cutting board
- ~ Sharp knife for cleaning pumpkin
- ~ Casserole for cooking pumpkin
- ~ Bowl for soaking raisins
- ~ Hinged baking pan, 24 cm in diameter
- ~ Baking paper
- ~ Saucepan for syrup
- ~ Latex gloves
- ~ Sieve

Preparation

First of all clean the pumpkin: remove filaments and internal seeds and deprive it of the hard and massive peel. Reduce the pulp into small pieces.

In the meantime prepare the syrup, which we will only need for the maceration of the apples. In a small saucepan, dissolve the brown sugar in boiling water. Let cool completely, first at room temperature, then in the refrigerator.

Soak the raisins in hot water for at least 10 minutes.

In a saucepan, heat 1 tablespoon of extra-virgin olive oil and sauté the pumpkin pulp. Add the softened raisins, well drained from the soaking water, and a pinch of salt. Cook until pureed.

In the meantime, cut the 2 apples (which we will need for decoration) into thin slices and leave them to macerate in the cooled syrup.

Peel the remaining apple and cut it into small pieces. Add the apple to the pumpkin pulp, now reduced to a cream.

In the same pot, add the whole-wheat flour and sifted baking powder.

Line a hinged baking pan with a diameter of 24 cm with baking paper and, with the help of hands greased with a tablespoon of oil, arrange the mixture. Arrange the apple slices, drained from the syrup, on the surface.

Bake the pumpkin and apple pie in a preheated oven at 200°C and bake for 15 minutes. After that, lower the temperature to 160°C and continue for another 35 minutes.

Remove the cake from the oven and cut when well chilled.

Simple Cake with Coconut Sugar

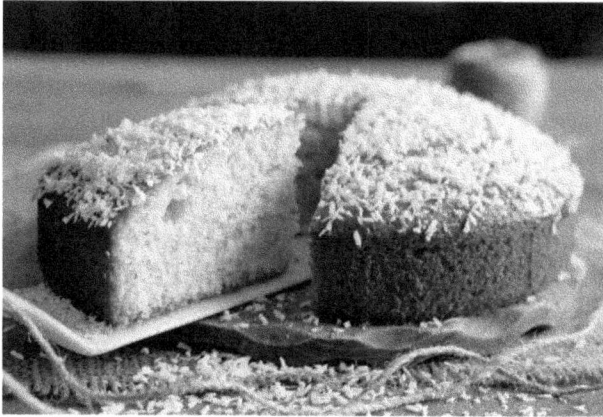

Recipe ID card

- ~ 216 Kcal calories per serving
- ~ Easy difficulty
- ~ Serves 8
- ~ Preparation 15 minutes
- ~ Average cost
- ~ 15 minutes for preparation; 35 minutes for cooking

Ingredients

- ~ 250 g of wholemeal flour
- ~ 1 pinch of salt
- ~ 20 g of bitter cocoa
- ~ Essence of vanilla
- ~ 300 g of pears
- ~ 60 ml of corn seed oil
- ~ 200 ml of milk
- ~ 120 g (2 egg whites + 2 yolks) of eggs
- ~ 100 g of coconut sugar
- ~ 10 g of baking powder

Material Required

- ~ Hinged baking pan with a diameter of 22 cm
- ~ Bowl
- ~ Electric whisk
- ~ Chopping board
- ~ Knife

Preparation

In a bowl, gather all dry ingredients: whole wheat flour, cocoa, coconut sugar, vanilla flavor and salt.

Shell the eggs and separate the yolks from the whites.

In the center, combine the milk, oil and yolks: mix the ingredients to obtain a thick cream.

Collect the egg whites in a bowl and whip them until stiff with electric whips. Add the frothy mass of egg whites to the mixture, taking care to mix the mixture slowly and from top to bottom to avoid sagging the mixture.

As a final ingredient, add the cake yeast and mix the powder into the other ingredients.

Pour the cream into a baking tin lined with baking paper with a diameter of 22 cm. Decorate the surface with pear segments, previously peeled.

Bake immediately and bake at 160°C (mode: ventilated) for 35-40 minutes or until the cake is perfectly cooked.

Cut into slices and serve. We recommend storing the cake in the refrigerator and consuming it within 3 days. Before serving the cake, we recommend reheating it quickly in the oven. For a sinful version, serve the pear and chocolate cake warm, accompanying it with a scoop of vanilla ice cream.

Simple Dukan Cake

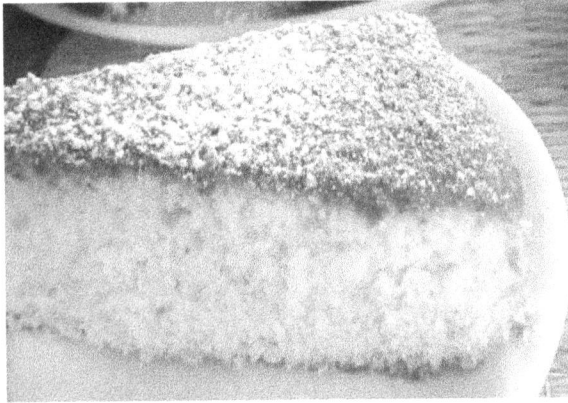

Recipe ID card

- ~ 270 Kcal calories per serving
- ~ Easy difficulty
- ~ Serves 20 people
- ~ Preparation 40 minutes
- ~ Average cost
- ~ 15 minutes for preparation; 25 minutes for cooking

Ingredients

- ~ 160 g (4 medium) egg white
- ~ 15 g of bitter cocoa
- ~ 150 g of oat bran
- ~ 25 drops of TIC sweetener or 120 g of erythritol
- ~ 1 teaspoon of baking powder
- ~ 20 g of cornstarch
- ~ 1 pinch of salt
- ~ 80 g (4 medium) egg yolks
- ~ 170 g of Greek yogurt

Material Required

- ~ Electric whips
- ~ Bowls
- ~ Wooden ladle
- ~ Spatula
- ~ Hinged baking pan with a diameter of 24 cm
- ~ Baking paper
- ~ Sieve
- ~ Precision scales

Preparation

In a bowl, combine all the dry ingredients, i.e. the oat bran, erythritol, sifted unsweetened cocoa, corn-starch and baking powder.

Peel the eggs and separate the yolks from the whites. Whip the egg whites until stiff, adding a pinch of fine salt.

In the meantime, mix the yolks and low-fat Greek yogurt with all the dry ingredients until you have a fairly thick cream.

Line a baking sheet with baking paper; alternatively, you can use a silicone mold.

Slowly mix the egg whites a few at a time into the cream, taking care to always mix from the top down to avoid sagging the mixture.

Pour the mixture into the baking tin and bake in a hot oven (180°C) for about 25 minutes.

Cake with Pumpkin and Sweet Potatoes

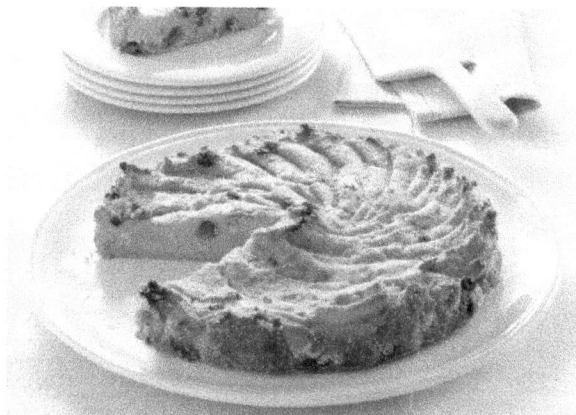

Recipe ID card

- ~ 211 Kcal calories per serving
- ~ Difficulty fairly easy
- ~ Serves 8
- ~ Preparation 30 minutes
- ~ Average cost
- ~ 30 minutes for preparation; 45 minutes for cooking

Ingredients

- ~ 200 g of pumpkin pulp
- ~ 1 sachet (16 g) of baking powder
- ~ 1 pinch of salt
- ~ 70 g of almonds
- ~ 80 ml of corn seed oil
- ~ 50 g of chickpea flour
- ~ 200 g of spelt
- ~ 200 ml of grape juice (recommended) or apple juice
- ~ 100 ml of soy milk
- ~ 200 g of sweet potatoes
- ~ 100 g of raisins

Material Required

- ~ Blender or grater
- ~ Hinged baking pan with a diameter of 24 cm
- ~ Baking paper
- ~ Bowl
- ~ Food scale
- ~ Food brush

Preparation

Clean the pumpkin. Wash the rind, dry it, cut the pumpkin in half, then remove the filaments and the internal seeds. Decorticate the pumpkin using a knife. Cut the pulp into cubes.

Wash the American potatoes, scrubbing the skin with a small food brush. Peel the sweet potatoes and cut them into small cubes.

Place and diced potatoes and squash in a blender and grind to a paste.

Blend almonds until a powder is obtained.

Grate the zest of one orange and squeeze out the juice. Soften the raisins in warm water.

Mix the chickpea flour with the soy milk to make a semi-liquid batter.

In a bowl, combine the chopped pumpkin and sweet potato, grape juice, squeezed raisins, corn oil and a pinch of salt. Combine the whole-wheat spelt flour, chickpea batter, chopped almonds, orange zest and juice and a packet of cake yeast.

Pour the mixture into a hinged mold with a diameter of 24 cm, lined with baking paper. Bake the cake in a hot oven, preheated to 160°C for 45 minutes.

Remove from the oven, allow to cool, cut into slices and serve.

Store in the refrigerator for 3-4 days.

Example Diet

<u>Retired lady who is able to take long walks. She takes hypoglycemic medications.</u>

Sex F

Age 77

Height 155 cm

Wrist circumference 15.5 cm

Constitution Normal

Height/wrist 10.0

Morphological type Normal

Weight kg 68

Body Mass Index 28.3

Assessment Overweight

Desirable physiological body mass index 21.7

Desirable Physiologic Weight kg   52,1

Basal metabolic rate kcal 1134.6

Physical activity level coefficient SI aus 1.56

Energy expenditure kcal 1769.9

Hypochaloric Diet -30% 1240 Kcal about

Lipids 30% 372kcal 41.3g

Protein 1.2g/kg * physiol. weight 250.1kcal 62.5g

Carbohydrates 50.0% 617.9kcal 164.8g

Breakfast 15% 186kcal

Snack 10% 124kcal

Lunch 35% 434kcal

Snack 10% 124kcal

Dinner 30% 372kcal

Note. The example diet that follows refers to a case of diabetes mellitus type 2 already pharmacologically compensated; therefore, the use of pasta and bread is allowed; however, even if glycemia would be higher, it would not be possible to excessively distort the nutritional balance of the diet in favor of fats (which would limit weight loss) and/or proteins (which could excessively fatigue the liver and kidneys of a subject in old age).

Example diet for Diabetes Type 2

DAY 1

Breakfast,	about 15%kcal TOT
Low-fat milk,	2% of total 150ml, 75.0kcal
Wholemeal bread, stale bread.	50g, 121,5kcal
Snack,	about 10%kcal TOT
Low-fat yogurt	125g, 70,0kcal
Strawberries	150g, 48,0kcal
Lunch,	about 35%kcal TOT
Pasta with tomato sauce	
Whole wheat pasta	80g, 259,2kcal
Tomato sauce	100g, 24,0kcal
Parmesan cheese	10g, 39,2kcal
Lettuce	100g, 18.0kcal
Extra virgin olive oil	15g, 135,0kcal
Snack,	about 10%kcal TOT
Low-fat yogurt	125g, 70,0kcal
Sour red cherries	100g, 50,0kcal
Dinner,	about 30%kcal TOT
Grilled chicken breast	
Chicken breast	100g, 110,0kcal
Eggplant	200g, 48,0kcal
Wholemeal bread	25g, 60,8kcal
Extra virgin olive oil	15g, 135.0kcal

DAY 2

Breakfast,	about 15%kcal TOT
Low-fat milk,	2% of total 150ml, 75.0kcal
Wholemeal bread, stale bread	50g, 121,5kcal
Snack,	about 10% kcal TOT
Low-fat yogurt	125g, 70,0kcal
½ orange	200g, 63,0kcal
Lunch,	about 35%kcal TOT
Stewed beans	
Dried beans	80g, 279,9kcal
Parmesan cheese	10g, 39,2kcal
Radicchio	100g, 24,0kcal
Extra virgin olive oil	15g, 135,0kcal
Snack,	about 10%kcal TOT
Low-fat yogurt	125g, 70,0kcal
½ orange	200g, 63,0kcal
Dinner,	about 30%kcal TOT
Trout fillet	
Trout, various species	100g, 148,0kcal
Fennel	200g, 62,0kcal
Wholemeal bread	25g, 60,8kcal
Extra virgin olive oil	10g, 90.0kcal

DAY 3

Breakfast,	about 15%kcal TOT
Low-fat milk,	2% of total 150ml, 75.0kcal
Wholemeal bread, stale bread	50g, 121,5kcal
Snack,	about 10%kcal TOT
Low-fat yogurt	125g, 70,0kcal
½ apple, with peel	200g, 52,0kcal
Lunch,	about 35%kcal TOT
Plain rice	
Brown rice	80g, 289,6kcal
Parmesan cheese	10g, 39,2kcal
Arugula	100g, 25,0kcal
Extra virgin olive oil	15g, 135,0kcal
Snack,	about 10%kcal TOT
Low-fat yogurt	125g, 70,0kcal
½ apple, with peel	200g, 52,0kcal
Dinner,	about 30%kcal TOT
Hard-boiled eggs	
Chicken grape	100g, 143,0kcal
Potato	100g, 85,0kcal
Wholemeal bread	25g, 60.8kcal
Extra virgin olive oil	5g, 45.0kcal

DAY 4

Breakfast,	about 15%kcal TOT
Low-fat milk,	2% of total 150ml, 75.0kcal
Wholemeal bread, stale bread	50g, 121,5kcal
Snack,	about 10%kcal TOT
Low-fat yogurt	125g, 70,0kcal
Kiwi	100g, 61,0kcal
Lunch,	about 35%kcal TOT
Chickpeas in broth	
Chickpeas, dried	90g, 300,6kcal
Parmesan cheese	10g, 39,2kcal
Valerian	100g, 18,0kcal
Extra virgin olive oil	15g, 135,0kcal
Snack,	about 10%kcal TOT
Low-fat yogurt	125g, 70,0kcal
Kiwi	100g, 61,0kcal
Dinner,	about 30%kcal TOT
Pan-fried cod fillet	
Atlantic cod fillet	100g, 82,0kcal
Swiss chard	200g, 38,0kcal
Whole wheat bread	25g, 60,8kcal
Extra virgin olive oil	15g, 135,0kcal

DAY 5

Breakfast,	about 15%kcal TOT
Low-fat milk,	2% of total 150ml, 75.0kcal
Wholemeal bread, stale bread	50g, 121,5kcal
Snack,	about 10%kcal TOT
Low-fat yogurt	125g, 70,0kcal
Strawberries	150g, 48,0kcal
Lunch,	about 35%kcal TOT
Eggplant pasta	
Whole wheat pasta	80g, 259,2kcal
Eggplant	100g, 24,0kcal
Parmesan cheese	10g, 39,2kcal
Lettuce	100g, 18.0kcal
Extra virgin olive oil	15g, 135,0kcal
Snack,	about 10%kcal TOT
Low-fat yogurt	125g, 70,0kcal
Sour red cherries	100g, 50,0kcal
Dinner,	about 30%kcal TOT
Turkey breast	
Chicken breast	100g, 111,0kcal
Zucchini	200g, 36,0kcal
Wholemeal bread	25g, 60,8kcal
Extra virgin olive oil	15g, 135.0kcal

DAY 6

Breakfast,	about 15%kcal TOT
Low-fat milk,	2% of total 150ml, 75.0kcal
Wholemeal bread, stale bread	50g, 121,5kcal
Snack,	about 10%kcal TOT
Low-fat yogurt	125g, 70,0kcal
½ orange	200g, 63,0kcal
Lunch,	about 35%kcal TOT
Stewed beans	
Dried beans	80g, 279,9kcal
Parmesan cheese	10g, 39,2kcal
Radicchio	100g, 24,0kcal
Extra virgin olive oil	15g, 135,0kcal
Snack,	about 10%kcal TOT
Low-fat yogurt	125g, 70,0kcal
½ orange	200g, 63,0kcal
Dinner,	about 30%kcal TOT
Trout fillet	
Trout, various species	100g, 97,0kcal
Fennel	200g, 62,0kcal
Wholemeal bread	25g, 60,8kcal
Extra virgin olive oil	15g, 135,0kcal

DAY 7

Breakfast,	about 15%kcal TOT
Low-fat milk,	2% of total 150ml, 75.0kcal
Wholemeal bread, stale bread	50g, 121,5kcal
Snack,	about 10%kcal TOT
Low-fat yogurt	125g, 70,0kcal
½ apple, with peel	200g, 52,0kcal
Lunch,	about 35%kcal TOT
Plain rice	
Brown rice	80g, 289,6kcal
Parmesan cheese	10g, 39,2kcal
Arugula	100g, 25,0kcal
Extra virgin olive oil	15g, 135,0kcal
Snack,	about 10%kcal TOT
Low-fat yogurt	125g, 70,0kcal
½ apple, with peel	200g, 52,0kcal
Dinner,	about 30%kcal TOT
Ricotta cheese	
Cow's milk ricotta, partially skimmed	100g, 138,0kcal
Endive	200g, 36,0kcal
Wholemeal bread	25g, 60,8kcal
Extra virgin olive oil	10g, 90,0kcal

APPENDIX

Cooking Conversion Charts

INGREDIENTS	CONVERSION US	CONVERSION EU
cup	16 tablespoons	236 ml
fluid ounce – fl.oz.	–	30 ml
pinch / dash	1/16 teaspoon	–
pint	2 cups	0,47 l
pound	16 ounces	454 g
quart	4 cups	0,95 l
teaspoon – tsp	1/3 tablespoon	5 ml
tablespoon – tbsp	3 teaspoons	15 ml
ounce – oz	–	28 g

Dry Ingredients

INGREDIENTS	CONVERSION
Cake/Pastry Flour	1 cup : 115 g
All-purpose	1 cup : 125 g
High gluten	1 cup : 140 g
Whole wheat	1 cup : 120 g
Bread flour	1 cup : 130 g
Spelt	1 cup : 100 g
Light Rye	1 cup : 100 g
Dark Rye	1 cup : 125 g
Buckweat	1 cup : 120 g
Rice	1 cup : 185 g
Sugar	1 cup : 200 g
Brown Sugar	1 cup : 220 g
Powdered Sugar	1 cup : 120 g
Baking Soda	1 tsp : 5 g
Baking Powder	1 tsp : 5 g
Fresh yeast	1 tsp : 3 g
Active dry yeast	1 tsp : 3 g
Salt	1 tbsp : 18 g
Chocolate chips	1 cup : 160 g
Cocoa	1 cup : 120 g

Fresh ingredients

INGREDIENTS	CONVERSIONS
Water	1 cup : 236 ml
Milk	1 cup : 245 ml
Yogurt	1 cup : 245 ml
Cream	1 cup : 245 ml
Buttermilk	1 cup : 245 ml
Olive Oil	• 1 cup : 222 ml • 1 tbsp : 13 g
Butter	• 1 cup : 230 g • 1 tbsp : 14.5 g • 1 stick : 1/2 cup : 8 tbsp : 115 g
Eggs	1 cup : 275 g
(Egg) Whites	1 cup : 240 g
(Egg) Yolks	1 cup : 300 g
Honey	• 1 cup : 340 g • 1 tbsp : 20 g
Grated cheese	1 cup : 110 g
Vanilla extract	1 tsp : 4 g
Peanut Butter	1 cup : 258 g

Oven Temperatures

250 °F	120 °C
275 °F	140 °C
300 °F	150 °C
325 °F	160 °C
350 °F	180 °C
375 °F	190 °C
400 °F	200 °C
425 °F	220 °C
450 °F	230 °C
475 °F	240 °C
500 °F	260 °C